ORGASM IN 5 MINUTES

1001 ROADS TO HAPPINESS

TINA ROBBINS

TRANSLATED BY
GLADIS CASTILLO

Skyhorse Publishing

T0016830

Skyhorse Publishing books may be purchased in bulk at special discounts
for sales promotion, corporate gifts, fund-raising, or educational purposes.
Special editions can also be created to specifications. For details, contact
the Special Sales Department, Skyhorse Publishing, 307 West 36th Street,
11th Floor, New York, NY 10018 or info@skyhorsepublishing.com.

Skyhorse® and Skyhorse Publishing® are registered trademarks of Skyhorse
Publishing, Inc.®, a Delaware corporation.

Visit our website at www.skyhorsepublishing.com.

10 9 8 7 6 5 4 3 2 1

Library of Congress Cataloging-in-Publication Data is available on file.

Cover design by Liz Driesbach
Cover photo credit Thinkstock

ISBN: 978-1-5107-7262-5
eBook ISBN: 978-1-63220-079-2

Printed in the United States of America

Contents

INTRODUCTION   **7**

WHAT ARE MY SEXUAL ORGANS LIKE? WHAT IS AN ORGASM?   **9**
STAGES OF AN ORGASM   11
BODY EXPLORATION   13
EXERCISES TO INCREASE CONTROL OVER YOUR SEXUALITY   14

SEX STARTS IN THE MIND   **17**
MISCONCEPTIONS   19
DO YOU CONSIDER YOURSELF ATTRACTIVE?   21
YOU ARE ATTRACTIVE!   23
MIND THE DETAILS...AND FLIRT   24
FLIRTING AND ORGASMS   26

MASTURBATION   **27**
THE CLITORIS   30
THE G-SPOT   30
THE URETHRA   31
EMOTIONAL AND ALTERNATIVE ORGASMS   31
SOME SUGGESTIONS   32
BENEFITS OF MASTURBATION   32
PROBLEMS?   33

Sex with a partner **37**
I also know how to fake it 40
The 10 most exciting positions 41
Helpful tips 49

Fantasies and orgasms are inseparable **51**
I do not know how to fantasize 53
How do I do it? 54
Should I share my fantasies with my partner? ... 56
Toys and stimuli 58

Guys, this is what we like! **65**
Some misconceptions 65
Some helpful tips 68
The appropriate sequence 71
Some concrete techniques 75

Sex and fear **77**
The ideal contraceptive method 77
Sexually transmitted diseases (STDs) 82

In depth **87**
Multiple orgasms 87
Simultaneous orgasms 89
Tantric orgasms 92
Anal sex 95
Variations and variants 97

Doubts, questions, and testimonials **101**
Doubts and questions 101
Some complaints 107
Testimonials 110

Now what? **113**

Glossary **117**

Introduction

The female orgasm is the most simple and natural thing in the world, but oftentimes we complicate this matter to the point of absurdity, as if it were something mysterious, intricate, or requiring special skills.

Have you ever heard of a man having trouble reaching an orgasm? I am not referring to people with serious physical conditions. I am talking about ordinary people like you and me, who want to have sex with their partner and enjoy it. For men, we are more used to hearing that their problem is that they have an orgasm "too fast," as if they were competing in a race.

Why should it be any different for women? The idea that men go on a Ferrari while we are merely on a bike when it comes to orgasms is completely false. Sexual attraction is perhaps the most powerful engine of life and nature; very wisely, it has determined that the sexes be attracted to guarantee the continuity of the species. They are attracted because their instinct tells them that they will enjoy the sexual union; that is, they are going to have an orgasm. This happens in all animal species without any qualms about it. Nor does it appear that, among humans, men have the least problem in this regard. So, what about women? Why should we have any difficulty? Is there something in our bodies that makes it harder for us to reach sexual climax? The answer is no. All women can have an orgasm every time they make love. And they can get to it pretty quickly...if they are interested.

The barriers that keep us from having orgasms are inherited prejudices given in a patriarchal society where for centuries female pleasure was regarded with suspicion, if not disapproval. Fortunately, in today's world, these prejudices are in clear decline, and women can openly claim the right to enjoy their bodies. Some information and a little practice is all you need to have an orgasm every time you make love. Whether you are single or married, divorced or widowed, whether you have had sexual experiences or not, whether you are shy or uninhibited, for you, reaching the climax will be as natural as eating if you are hungry, or drinking if you are thirsty.

In this book you will find all the information you need, along with exercises, tips, and techniques to enjoy sex and make your partner enjoy it, too. Leave behind your fears and your doubts! And dare to know the thousand and one ways to an orgasm...and to happiness.

Note: "In 5 minutes?" It is likely that the title of the book (designed to attract attention) has aroused your skepticism. For one thing, when there is something we like, we like it to last much more than 5 minutes. For another, it would seem contradictory to publish books on Tantra (ecstatic sexual practice that includes orgasms without ejaculation, which usually lasts several hours) next to this one you have in your hands.

The truth is that it is not simple to incorporate Tantra (which in the East is something sacred and a form of meditation) into daily life. It is not too easy to connect with like-minded people who enjoy the same availability of time and share the right frame of mind that allows us to live the tantric experience in a usual way. So, although the recommendations in this book may seem more modest, we believe that they will be useful for everyone and are not intended to rule out such a noble path. And bear in mind, along with the poet, that in one way or another, "for those who love, time is eternity." Enjoy it!

What are my sexual organs like? What is an orgasm?

"When I talk to friends about my sexual experiences, and I tell them that I don't always have an orgasm because it seems to depend on my partner's skill, they always insist on the importance of the clitoris. They say that's where the secret lies because it's pleasurable to have it touched... And I'm ashamed to admit to them that I don't know where it is."

Julia, 24 years old

The first step to reaching an orgasm easily and quickly is to know your body. There is widespread evidence that the female orgasm is caused by direct or indirect stimulation of the clitoris, the same way that the male orgasm occurs through stimulation of a particular area of the glans penis. So, it is not surprising that some women have difficulty reaching an orgasm through penetration alone: the penis fails to touch the clitoris, and that makes it difficult. Imagine how it would be for a man to reach an orgasm simply by having his testicles caressed. He would never get there, or it would take him forever.

That is the issue. There is no such thing as a delay; what happens is that due to ignorance, many times the correct area is not stimulated and the orgasm takes a while.

Knowing your vagina, the exact location of the clitoris, the urethra, and the arrangement of the inner and outer lips will help you a lot in achieving your goals.

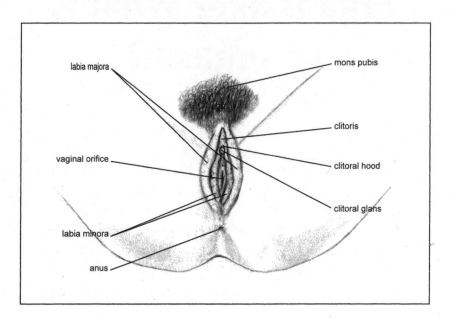

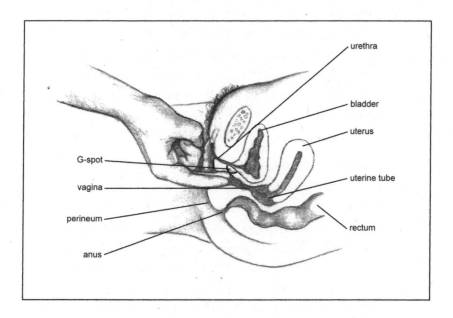

STAGES OF AN ORGASM

Having that knowledge from the start will allow you to explore your own body and discover which type of stimulation, posture, and caresses excite you the most. The majority of women have their first orgasm alone in a relaxed and calm manner when they explore their genital area. Later we will give precise instructions on how you should do this. First, and to continue with this brief physiology lesson, we will describe the stages your body goes through when you reach an orgasm:

1. **Excitement.** After kissing and cuddling with your partner for a while, you probably notice that a sensation of emptiness takes over your body. This is the beginning of the sexual cycle, called "awakening." The heart starts to pump a little faster, the breasts seem to swell and the nipples harden, the blood flow rushes into the pelvis, the uterus contracts, and the labia swell slightly and begin to secrete lubricating fluids.

2. **Plateau.** This phase is much less noticeable because almost everything happens inside your body. The vagina increases in size, the labia minora darken and open slightly, and the uterus moves up: your body gets ready to receive sperm. At the same time, you feel blood rushing through your veins at galloping speeds.

3. **Climax.** Blood flows into the breasts, and they are enlarged even further. Breathing becomes more rapid and agitated, to the point that you may moan. The big moment has arrived! The clitoris becomes erect, and too much friction can be a bit bothersome. The labia swell. The muscles of the vagina contract spasmodically between three and seven times, as a kind of electric shock producing an intense sensation of pleasure. The anus contracts, and your heartbeat and breathing intensify.

4. **Resolution.** In this last stage of the cycle, the body returns to normal. The blood flows away from the pelvis, the breasts regain their normal size, and there is a general feeling of satisfaction and fulfillment. The heart rate lowers, and the uterus and vagina return to their normal shape and size. The increased blood pressure in the previous stages will give your cheeks a rosy pink color.

Perhaps the best way for you to really get to know your sexual organs, how the different parts are arranged, and what forms of stimulation you find easier and more enjoyable is by using the sense of touch. Touch plays a crucial role in the enjoyment of sexual sensations. If you familiarize yourself with your genitals by touch, it will be much easier to subtly direct another person's touch to where you actually experience pleasure. We will suggest a few simple exercises for you to try on your genital area until you familiarize yourself with it. The purpose of this book is not to present complicated technical descriptions of your sexual organs. Instead, we intend to show a simple and practical way to discover yourself, to learn about your body, and to enjoy it. Practicing this exercise may help you find that very intense orgasm you want.

BODY EXPLORATION

Lie down comfortably in a place where you are safe from prying eyes. Bend your knees and open your legs a bit.

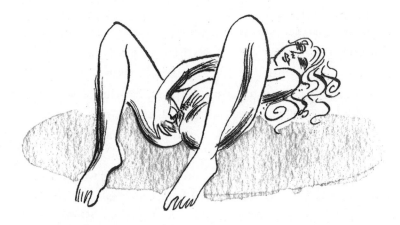

Start by gently exploring all your body parts: arms, breasts, abdomen, and inner thighs. Touch yourself in different ways: using your fingertips, the palms of your hands, and your wrists, perhaps.

Change positions whenever you want and become acquainted with your curves and angles, as well as with the hard and soft parts of your body.

Gently explore your pubic hair, labia majora (or outside of your vagina), and perineum muscle that is between your vagina and anus.

Slide your fingertips along the inner or outer labia and the urethra, and continue upward to locate the clitoris.

Explore your clitoris carefully. Check to see if you can feel it through the clitoral hood covering. Move around the clitoral hood and gently touch it.

Place your fingers down the outside of the vaginal opening, and insert one or two fingers gently, until you feel your wet warmth.

Push your fingers further inside until you find the "G-spot," which is located about an inch inside the wall of the vagina. You will notice it because it is a small, particularly sensitive bump.

To wrap things up, go back to exploring other areas of your body, **take a deep breath**...and go to the fridge and grab something you enjoy, like a tomato juice or a yogurt.

Practice this exercise several times until you feel that you "know" your body—you know where everything is and what texture it all is. You will see how this will be very useful for the next steps that we will suggest for you to have an orgasm. Sexuality is a complex phenomenon involving many factors: education, culture, religion, social conventions, feelings, and passions...accumulations of external things that largely determine the type of relationship that people, especially women, have with sex. In this book you will encounter responses and behavior patterns to help you break free from the external prejudices imposed on you, and bring you closer to your sexuality in a more natural, simple, and pleasant way!

When sexual sensations start taking over your body, whether you are alone or with your partner, your muscles, organs, and body parts come into play, and it is important to recognize them and, to some extent, control them to achieve things the way you want.

Exercises to increase control over your sexuality

Now, a few simple exercises to learn to identify and feel aspects of your body that are essential to having sex: breathing, breasts, pelvis, and vagina.

Inhaling and exhaling. The breathing rate varies with the emotional state. Throughout foreplay, prior to an orgasm, breathing adapts to each of the phases that the body goes through: excitement, plateau, climax, and resolution. It is important to breathe smoothly throughout this process, because if the breathing rate is inadequate, your excitement could potentially keep you from reaching the culminating point. Initially, try to keep your breathing deep and balanced to help your body relax. Keep your mouth slightly open, and as you inhale allow your lungs and stomach to swell a little. Always make sure not to hold your breath, because this can cause tension that is very counterproductive to the full enjoyment of your physical sensations.

Breast exercises. Do you like to caress your breasts? Do you notice that in doing so your blood flow accelerates and a slight tingling appears in your genital area? Sure! Relaxation in this part of the body is essential for sexual enjoyment. Lie down on your back and take a deep breath. Raise your arms over your head, forming an arc. As you breathe out, put your arms back down. Repeat this five times. Then do the opposite: raise your arms to breathe out and then lower them as you inhale. Five more times. Do you feel a slight tingling in the arms and face? Enjoy that feeling, because it is similar to that tingling sensation after having an orgasm.

Balancing and pelvic thrusts. The movements of this exercise are similar to penetration and masturbation. Lie down on your back with your knees bent and your feet touching the mattress or carpet. Lift your hips and pelvis up and down. To raise your body more easily, push off with your hands.

Vaginal exercises. Do you feel the muscles in your vagina? Are you aware that they are important for sex? The vaginal muscles should be exercised just like the rest of the body. It has been shown that by increasing the strength of these muscles, orgasms are more likely and more intense—first, because it increases blood flow to that area of the body; second, because the genitals gain strength, and that increases the chances of having an orgasm.

Initially, these are muscles that one "does not feel," just like the stomach or bowels. However, with a little practice you will come to feel and control them. Can you imagine the pleasure you can experience when you notice that the muscles around your vagina surround and push your partner's penis? Simply focus your mind on your vagina and try to contract and relax the muscles in that area. This is a similar movement we make to hold urine when there is no bathroom nearby. At first you can contract and count to three, then relax. Do not worry if the first few times you do not notice anything. With a little practice you will notice your muscles, you will feel as they contract and relax, and you get to control them more easily.

It will require a little extra concentration only at the beginning. Then everything will be a breeze, and you can practice anywhere because nobody will notice. You can do it while lying, standing, sitting, or reclining. On the bus, at work, leaning at a bar: only you will be aware that you are contracting and relaxing the muscles of your vagina and preparing to fully enjoy sex...when the time comes.

Sex starts in the mind

"Women with confidence are so sexy! I cannot stand women who hate their bodies, or just talk about their flaws, or constantly complain. To be honest, I only notice women who show themselves as they are. A woman who likes herself is always attractive."

Jaime, 38 years old

Some say that true sexual activity happens in the mind...and the rest is pure gymnastics. I am not sure that is true. We have already seen how other parts of the body respond to sex very precisely. However, are you able to let go? Do you tremble at the thought of surrendering completely? Are you one of those people who cannot "lose control" for a minute? To have an orgasm, it is essential that you let go, surrender, and lose control. You also need to put aside any stress. But for some of us that is difficult. If that is your case, do not worry. You are just average. How many times have we heard, since an early age, that girls do not touch themselves, that they should not show their legs? How many times have we been told to be careful around boys because they are only after "one thing"? Everything we have been taught for generations about sex is very imprinted on our minds, and it is not easy to act naturally if our minds are full of all that trash!

In this chapter, I will tell you what you have to do to see yourself as a sexual being who feels sensual and wants to enjoy sex—to see yourself as someone who wants to have orgasms and enjoy her body. Because it is natural, because it is healthy, and because you deserve it.

To have an orgasm, you must see yourself as an orgasmic person. To be attractive, you have to feel attractive. Do you know anyone, man or woman, who is always attractive? Can you stand that individual? Is his or her arrogance insufferable? Typically you feel sexy sometimes, and other times you will be disappointed by your reflection in the mirror; you like your hair or your waist or your chest, but not every single part of your body. No one can expect to always feel like Miss Universe. The important thing is that you feel like a sexual person who attracts and is attracted to your partner, and that you accept this as something logical, natural, and positive, no matter how you were raised. This is not the time to berate your parents or educators who instilled those ideas in you. It is time to act. You are an adult. You are free. You can decide. You want to enjoy sex? Want to have orgasms alone or with someone? Are you willing to accept that thoughts about sex are not "bad"? If that is your decision, go for it! Reading this book will help you achieve those goals.

The first and most important step is to make a decision. Plainly. *I want to have orgasms! I want to enjoy sex! Sex is clean, natural, and good for my body and my mind! I deserve to enjoy it, and I deserve orgasms and pleasure!* If this decision is not final, if you keep mulling over the idea that sex is bad or wrong or inappropriate for women, your body will express that fear, that indecision, that barrier...and others will notice.

But that is not your case! You have decided to be a sexual person and enjoy your body whenever you feel like it! Bravo, that is the way to go! Continue reading, and you will not have even the slightest doubt that you will achieve this.

Misconceptions

Some of the notions that follow have been heard many times in conversations with friends or in comments between people at work. They are part of the huge amount of prejudice that relates to female sexuality. Beware! None of them have anything to do with reality. They are in response to an old and outdated conception of sex and women. You have decided to be a sexual person and want to have orgasms easily. It will not hurt you to remember some of the most common fallacies that are ignorantly repeated, so that you can turn a deaf ear to them the next time you hear them say:

Sex is for those under 30. If you are younger than that, this does not affect you, but if you are older... Forget this nonsense! There is widespread evidence that sexual responsiveness in women increases with age. In your 30s you are at the peak of your sexual prowess. Afterward, too! Only disease is responsible for a significant decline in sexual interest and activity.

A decent woman does not get aroused by erotic articles. Can you imagine Brad Pitt caressing you tenderly? I consider myself to be very "decent," and I confess that the thought turns me on. Do "decent" men get excited by their favorite actress or by an erotic movie? Excitement that stems from fantasies, erotic images, or readings has absolutely nothing to do with decency or gender. Human beings get aroused by certain images, but, again, the degree of arousal as a response to these stimuli depends on each person.

"FEMININE" WOMEN DO NOT TAKE THE INITIATIVE DURING SEX

But are there "masculine" women? Women, all women, have desires and spontaneous impulses during sexual activity and take the initiative if they want. It is rather a matter of character and personality that is applicable to both men and women. If you like taking the initiative, do not hesitate for a moment. The idea that men prefer "passive" women is just another prejudice. But do not obsess over initiating. Just act according to your own personality.

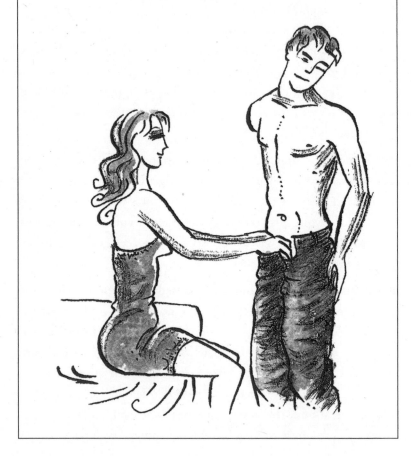

If a woman does not like certain forms of sex, she is frigid. Please! If you do not like swinging, oral or anal sex, or orgies, you are just like millions of women worldwide. Sex is something very personal, and not everyone likes the same things. Enjoy what you like and forget the rest.

A woman without erotic fantasies is lascivious; the one without them is frigid. Fortunately, imagination is free. Every person can have the sexual fantasies that they crave. They are part of your privacy that is absolutely unbreakable, and have nothing to do with morality, nor the sexual responsiveness of each person. If a specific fantasy helps you have a more intense orgasm, do not deprive yourself! Your partner cares much more about you enjoying yourself than finding out what you are thinking. And if his curiosity proves to be too much, just lie! Nobody has the right to breach your innermost thoughts.

There are different types of orgasms. Vaginal orgasms are more feminine than clitoral orgasms. An orgasm is an orgasm. The ways to describe them vary because, as the poets say, the ineffable is difficult to express. But the feelings of intense pleasure, the uncontrolled contractions of the uterus, and the feeling of fullness are just what they are. If you orgasm by stroking your clitoris while in the shower, you are as feminine as Lady Di, and you also know how to enjoy your body.

Do you consider yourself attractive?

"I could never agree to have sex in front of a mirror because all I would see was my huge, flabby ass. But one day my partner started telling me that my skin was soft, smooth, and desirable. Since then, my focus is on this aspect of my body, and in the mirror I see a much more attractive image of myself."

Susana, 29 years old

You have already decided to be a sexual person. Now you have to do something to convince yourself that your responsiveness and your sex appeal are at a more reasonable level. Perhaps you have had enough experience for this issue to not present a problem for you. In which case, that is even better! But maybe your confidence is lacking more than necessary. It is possible that when you look in the mirror in the nude, you see nothing more than breasts that are too big or too small, or cellulite thighs, or hipbones, and that makes you feel unattractive and undesirable. I once read a self-help book that said the solution was for me to repeat this to myself in front of the mirror: "I'm sexy, I'm sexy, and I'm sexy." The result was the same as when I repeated for weeks, "I'm rich, I'm rich, I'm rich," and I still had a hard time making ends meet. One day, a male friend told me that a naked woman is always attractive to a man, because when you are in bed with a lover, he is not evaluating the amount of cellulite on your buttocks or your stretch marks, what he sees and what he thinks is "breasts, ass, bare skin, yummy!" He is looking at your naked body and thinking about sex, and then he is not too worried about small or large breasts, or hipbones.

Later I was able to confirm through my own experience that what my friend told me was absolutely true: at that moment, men only care that there is a naked woman. If you are naked in front of him and wanting to have sex, you will really feel attractive and desirable. If that is not the case, you better leave. If all he expects is that you should feel grateful that someone like him is with you, it means that he is someone who does not deserve you, and it is not worth it for you to invest your time, your energy, and your attractiveness.

But the issues that most often affect sexual confidence in women have to do with feelings of guilt and fear. The education that these women receive is so rigorous, close-minded, and macho, in this sense, that it is not easy for a woman to free herself from the many prejudices and preconceptions that were instilled in her during her lifetime, and those before her for generations. What to do when one feels gripped by guilt at the mere fact of feeling sexual desire? How to combat this unbearable feeling of guilt that overwhelms us after having casual sex?

If these inhibitions are rooted in some unfortunate experience in childhood or early adolescence, the only thing I can advise is for you to seek the help of a sex therapist. But if all those castrating ideas are merely the byproduct of your education, or what was instilled in you as a child, or through your friends' comments, my advice is simply to have more sex. There is a popular saying: "Wine is the best cure"; in this case we could change it to something like "Fear of sex is cured with more sex." You may need to start with some emotional support. If that is your case, it is best that you practice all your sexual encounters in a more or less stable, loving relationship.

Take gradual steps with your partner, enjoy new positions, practice the masturbation exercises you will find in this book, increase control over your vaginal muscles, know your body more and more, and find out what you like and what you dislike. You deserve it as a woman, and the result you will achieve is certainly worth it.

YOU ARE ATTRACTIVE!

The best and perhaps the only way you get to actually be an attractive and sexy woman is for you to live like one—no matter your age or marital status, and whether or not you have any luck with your partner. The truth is that everyone wants to be attractive to others, even to those people we do not like. If you want to become an attractive and desirable woman, you have no choice but to act as if you were already so. I am sure that you already are, but if you are still unconvinced, try to imagine how an attractive woman would act, and behave as she would.

The issue is to take action, not remain in this melancholic idea of "if I were like so-and-so... " You are equal to or better than so-and-so!

Just act the right way. If you think that a particular haircut or a certain nail color is very attractive, run to the hairdresser! If you feel that a slightly shorter skirt would enhance your knees, grab the scissors immediately! Imagine a party where a girl is sitting in a corner, sullenly, with her arms and legs crossed and looking at the ground, while another delicately stands by the doorway with her legs slightly open, looking around her with interest and smiling a little while making eye contact with others. Which of the two do you find more attractive, sexier, and more interesting? The answer is clear, don't you think? So, what are you doing sitting in the corner? Get up, smile, and do not cross your arms. If you act in a certain way, something will change in your brain, and you will really become a different person. It is not enough for you to repeat to yourself that you are attractive; doing that can help...but not much. If you really want to be attractive, sexy, exciting, sexually capable, and confident, you have to act like it. The results will surprise you. The truth is that we are all attractive, interesting, and sexy; what happens is that our inhibitions, fears, guilt, and such block us much more than we realize. Act as if none of these barriers exist for you and, in no time, notice how men start to flirt around you and you become an irresistible woman.

"Laughter is one of the sexiest things I know. I saw my current partner in a pub laughing uproariously. She looked so happy, and conveyed a sense of freedom so big! I immediately told myself I had to meet her."

Pablo, 34 years old

MIND THE DETAILS...AND FLIRT

You have already decided to act like a sexy and attractive woman, and you are not willing to shy away from this attempt. Do not ignore any details. Your hair can be a powerful point of attraction, provided it is clean and smooth; well-cared-for black eyelashes, nails polished in a color you like, or not at all, your apparel, shoes, handbag, belt—everything plays a role and must all be taken into account. This does not mean that you spend 3 hours a day in front of the mirror before you go out. You should never fall prey to exaggeration or affectation. It is simply a matter of taking care of the details of your appearance, but in a natural and "casual" way. Do not forget that first impressions are everything, and you should never exaggerate. Look into the eyes of others, but without insistence, smile, do not cross your arms ostensibly...with ease and confidence, as someone who knows her worth and is willing to share it...with someone worthwhile.

Whether you are married or have a steady partner, or whether you are single and without commitment, caring for yourself, both in the clothing you wear and the attitude you present to others, is very important. In both cases, acting with self-confidence in your own attractiveness and the way you are will not only increase the quality of your sexual life, if you are already sexually active, but it could also open up more doors than you can possibly imagine if you still do not have a partner. Flirting is essential in the life of a woman. But flirting does not mean making direct eye contact with whomever passes by first and asking that you get together. It is about keeping an open, warm, and friendly attitude toward those around us. Eye contact plays a fundamental role in the art of flirting. Look at your partner's face. Don't look directly in his eyes, because you could intimidate him. As if you were a painter, grace softly with your eyes the triangle formed between the outer ends of the eyebrows and his chin—without much insistence, yet sweetly. If you are very shy, this will not be too much of an effort, because you do not have to maintain eye contact with the other person. Just walk that magical space experts call "the triangle of seduction." You will always give the impression of being very interested not only in what you are hearing, but also in from whom you are hearing it.

People need to feel valued, heard, and appreciated. Through this simple and subtle way, you will create an atmosphere of trust and attraction with the person who is with you, regardless of whether it is your partner, someone at the office, or the old man you come across on the street when you go to buy bread. It is about keeping that attitude and making it yours, and it will become a part of you. If you get used to doing so, you will see that something changes within you, and that others, not just men, will notice.

FLIRTING AND ORGASMS

You are probably wondering what all this has to do with orgasms. Does wearing a shorter or longer skirt, having a particular haircut, or keeping an open and warm attitude toward others help you have an orgasm? The resounding answer is YES! Distrusting yourself, obsessing over your apparent physical defects, having a limited body language, and thinking you are not attractive, that you are not sexy, all are traps of your own mind that, although in the beginning you may not think so, can sometimes be insurmountable obstacles to getting to that deep and intense orgasm you want.

Enjoying sex, like enjoying life, is for people convinced that they deserve to. The care and attention to the details of your appearance, an open and friendly attitude toward others, and a sincere and confident body language are clear signs of a person who appreciates what is valuable, who knows she is attractive, and is able to enjoy what life offers. And, of course, someone who wants and knows how to enjoy sex.

You already know your body in detail and have the proper mental attitude to have sexual adventures. Read on and find all the secrets and keys to finding the satisfaction you seek.

Masturbation

"The pleasure that I get from orgasms varies depending on whether I am alone or with a man. When I am alone, I concentrate on stimulating my clitoris, and I orgasm much faster with a special intensity. I try to imagine the most exciting fantasy; then as I touch my clitoris, with increasing force, I feel myself reaching an orgasm. My body tenses, at times my breathing almost stops, the speed of the strokes increases, sometimes almost wildly, and, suddenly, wow! A rapid and intense spasm starts at my genitals and goes through my body. Then I feel a deep relaxation."

Marta, 27 years old

"I had never touched myself. At least not consciously. I thought it was very difficult. Not that I saw it as a 'sin,' but I did consider it as something wrong. Fortunately, I overcame my inhibitions, and I realized that I had never before had an orgasm. Now I know what I need, and what an orgasm means. I also know what I have to do to have it when I'm alone or if I'm with my partner."

Ana, 35 years old

For many women, it is difficult to admit that we masturbate. We are used to hearing that masturbation "is a man's thing" or that women cannot masturbate because they have no penis to touch, or it is "bad" or at least "an inappropriate habit for females." Nonsense!

The best way to convince you that masturbation is something nice, pleasurable, and even good for your health, is for you to put it into practice. In this chapter I will teach you to masturbate, in case you do not know how, or to improve your technique if you have been practicing for a while.

The benefits of masturbation, so that you will be the one controlling the speed and intensity of your orgasms, are innumerable. If you practice regularly, you will learn to "take the reins" during sex, regardless of whether your partner is an expert or not. The goal is to not depend on your partner to reach an orgasm, and for climax to be something so natural in your relationships that you can concentrate on other aspects of the sexual relationship, and you will not have to be worried beforehand, wondering, "Will I have an orgasm or won't I?" This assurance will free you from the fears that many women tend to have before sexual contact, it will make you feel more secure, and you will become much more attractive and interesting to others.

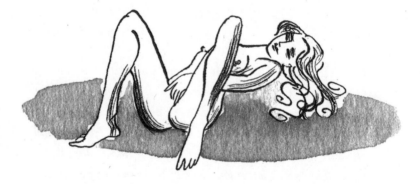

"With the fingers of one hand, hold the lips of your vagina open and stretched upwards. With the other hand, begin to gently caress your clitoris. With the skin stretched, the feeling is much more intense."

María, 32 years old

Have you been convinced of the importance and benefits of masturbation? So, let us practice. How do I masturbate? What is the best position? Should I use just my hands or use any device? Is it necessary for me to insert something into my vagina? The general answer to all these questions would be that you can do whatever you like or feel like at the time. If you prefer to use only your hands, perfect! If the idea of doing it while watching an erotic film excites you, no problem! If you tremble with excitement just thinking about your vagina getting penetrated by some kind of dildo, do not deprive yourself! It is essential that you banish from your mind any "bad" or "inconvenient" idea: masturbation is perfectly natural and healthy, and there should be nothing stopping you from enjoying your body as you want. Sitting, standing, lying down, while you shower, before bed, waking up... Any time is perfect to enjoy!

I will give you a short guide on the types of masturbation that most women find more pleasant. But do not forget that when it comes time to enjoy it, there are no limits other than those imposed by your own imagination.

The best position for you to masturbate depends much on the body part where you decide to focus. Normally, you will tend to focus on the clitoris, but it does not necessarily need to be so; there are other intensely erotic areas of the body that can also make you orgasm. In fact, ideally you should combine the stimulation of several parts at once.

> *"I mostly like to do it in bed, lying on my side. I run one of my hands behind my thigh, I put two fingers in my vagina, and I begin to gently move them in and out. With the other hand I touch my clitoris with increasingly rapid circular movements. I feel like an irresistible energy begins to circulate through every nerve in my body until...Ahhh!"*
>
> Penélope, 20 years old

The clitoris

Rest the base of the palm of your right hand in the pubic area, right where the hair starts. Place the tip of the clitoris between your middle and index fingers and gently begin to move up and down. With your other hand, stretch up the outer lips of the vagina while keeping them together. Try not to over-tighten the clitoris between your fingers. The pressure should be gentle as your body prompts you to speed up the movement. Do not forget that this is a very sensitive area, and if you push too hard, you may find it bothersome.

A variant of this technique is to insert one or two fingers of the left hand in your vagina, just a little, and make soft and delicate circular movements. This way you will stimulate all the nerves of the vaginal opening, which are also very sensitive. Any position can be good for this type of stimulation: lying with your knees slightly bent and your thighs slightly parted seems more normal. But why not try it standing, leaning against a wall, or in the shower?

Clitoral stimulation can be actually done in as many ways as you can imagine. I have a friend who does it while pedaling a bicycle! Her teammates have never understood why she is so fond of the sport. Another common way is to lie face down with your legs together and rub the pelvis against a cushion or pillow. The effect is the same: clitoral stimulation. In this case it is not so direct, and it will probably take longer to orgasm... It all depends on the time at your disposal!

Any of these techniques may be preceded or accompanied by caressing your breasts, inner thighs, or other body parts you enjoy touching.

The G-spot

This small protrusion, located about an inch inside the anterior vaginal wall, is especially sensitive, and some women I know would not change the sensation they experience when caressing it for anything else in the world. But in this case, a certain position is required, because it is not very easy to access this darned spot.

Lie on your back and bend your knees completely. Insert two fingers in the vagina facing toward the front, close to the belly. Three or four inches from it, you will notice a small bump on the skin, more or less the size of a penny. If you press firmly but without violence, you will notice that something like an erection happens: it gets a little harder and it seems to swell. That is the time to start to touch it while maintaining pressure on it. The feeling that awaits you is indescribable!

THE URETHRA

I know some women who find a special pleasure when they stimulate their urethra. This is the orifice where urine exits, which is located between the vagina and the clitoris. The technique involves stroking in a circular motion and always maintaining a certain pressure. Not all women reach an orgasm this way, but some have told me that if you combine touching the urethra with clitoral stimulation, the orgasm is much more intense.

EMOTIONAL AND ALTERNATIVE ORGASMS

An orgasm is not always preceded by stimulation of the genital area. Every woman, every person, is different. My female and male friends have orgasms by caressing their chests or by stimulating their anuses. It is even possible to get there using only your imagination, without any touching at all. Certainly it seems unlikely at first, but there are people capable of doing just that. In any case, it is ideal to combine the stimulation of at least two body parts to achieve more complete and more intense alternative orgasms. For example, you can try to caress your clitoris while pressing the G-spot, or caress your breasts or anus while moving your fingers up and down on the clitoral hood.

SOME SUGGESTIONS

The use of lubricants. Lubricating substances increase sensitivity and provide pleasure. It does not matter if they are vaginal secretions, artificial lubricants, or saliva. The only thing to keep in mind is that the genital skin is very sensitive, and some products can irritate. To avoid this, always use alcohol-free and water-based lubricants. Having said that, everything that contributes to increase sensitivity can facilitate an orgasm, so welcome it! Saliva is a natural substance that can prove to be extremely erotic. Play with it, and do not limit yourself.

Explore other textures and sensations. Try rubbing your body with a piece of velvet or a silk scarf—perhaps with a soft cotton towel. Anything that develops your creativity and inventiveness will improve your sex life and ease your orgasms. Experimenting with new sensations is the best prevention against routine and boredom.

The time to practice. Anytime can be a good time for an orgasm. However, sometimes the menstrual cycle may have some influence. It has been scientifically proven that around the eighteenth day of the cycle, your body is specially prepared to reach an orgasm. At that time of the month, your body produces extra amounts of pheromones that will make you more sexually aroused and attract the men around you. This hormone comes out through sweat and creates a very sexy aura around you. Seize the moment!

BENEFITS OF MASTURBATION

Masturbation is highly recommended by therapists and sexologists as the best way to show women that satisfaction does not just depend on men.

Women who masturbate regularly to reach an orgasm have no trouble achieving full sexual satisfaction in their relationships.

The same thing cannot be said of those who never or rarely masturbate.

The ability to have an orgasm through masturbation every time you want will greatly help keep up your self-esteem, boost your confidence, and increase your personal charm.

Masturbation is an excellent exercise for blood circulation, which helps improve the functioning of the cardiovascular system.

There is no better cure for stress than the regular practice of masturbation. The release of endorphins, brought on by an orgasm, is the best remedy for anxiety caused by the stress of modern life.

Whenever you touch your vagina and you have an orgasm, you are exercising and learning to understand and control the muscles in your genital area. This exercise will help prevent risks and complications during childbirth.

In the age of AIDS and all kinds of STDs, it is difficult to find a better way to practice safe sex.

PROBLEMS?

Maybe you have been practicing what we suggested, and the results have not been entirely satisfactory. I mean, you have a good time, but not enough. You have not been able to get to that high discharge, those sublime uncontrollable contractions that take you to seventh heaven. Do not despair, and do not get nervous. Maybe you were too tense or too relaxed, or your mind was elsewhere. We will give an overview of the most common situations that often occur to women who have a hard time achieving an orgasm while masturbating.

Too many expectations. So many of you have spent the entire time holding your breath. If you are in such a rush to reach an orgasm that you barely breathe, you may not get there. Remember what we told you in the previous chapter. Practice the exercises that we suggested. Your breathing should be deep and harmonious, and if not forced, it will adapt to each of the different phases.

Too much tension. Are you afraid that someone might walk in on you? Is it difficult for you to relax? Find a time of day exclusively for yourself. Lock the door, put a soft light on, and turn off the phone. Begin practicing the breathing exercise we indicated in the previous chapter and...enjoy!

Too much relaxation. Do you not get aroused? Does your body feel heavy and not respond? Maybe you are one of those women who need to put a little more excitement into the matter. Many of us feel much more excited in risky or unusual situations. I have a friend who likes it most in the elevator—she lives on the tenth floor—or while driving to work—I always tell her to pay attention to the road. Do not be shy! Try it on the subway or when you go to the bathroom at coffee time!

Friction bothers me. Surely it is because you are not sufficiently lubricated. The friction that occurs between your fingers and genital areas requires adequate lubrication. Remember the suggestions we made. If the vaginal fluid is not enough—do you insert your fingers in your vagina?—use saliva or an artificial lubricant that does not contain alcohol or aggressive substances.

I am unable to focus. Is your head always somewhere else? You have to make an effort to concentrate. You are having sex, and your mind should focus on that. Are you unable to get there? Use some external stimulus. How about a movie? Better yet, a book? Statistics show that women get more excited by words and pictures than men do. Do you agree? You can try with *Lady Chatterley's Lover* by D. H. Lawrence.

Blame it on your period. Remember that the menstrual cycle may influence your ability to reach an orgasm. Usually between the tenth and eighteenth day, the hormone levels in your body are at their peak. Those are days of increased fertility and sexual desire, so why not give it a try? During the days immediately before and after menstruation, there are many women who cannot even hear any talk about sex.

Take courage, friends! Masturbate in bed, in the bathroom, in the car. Do it whenever you have the chance. All women, including you, can have an orgasm, or more, whenever they want. Statistics show that women who masturbate regularly reach an orgasm in 3 to 5 minutes. And that is from the start, meaning without prior stimulation or an especially appropriate situation. Can you imagine how long it would take if you were previously aroused by some fantasy, or in the company of a gorgeous and desirable guy? If you still have not been able to get there in that time, it is simply for lack of practice. Explore your body, touch yourself, and learn what gives you pleasure. If you practice and practice, you will undoubtedly succeed.

Sex with a partner

"The union between a man and a woman is like Heaven and Earth mating. It is because of this correct mating that Heaven and Earth endure forever."

Chinese proverb

You have learned how to enjoy your body. You know how to reach an orgasm easily and without an hour-long effort. But as the proverb you just read suggests, the union with a man is like being in heaven. Experiencing an orgasm while making love with the person with whom you have chosen to share that moment is really something delicious and unique. The physical sensation of an orgasm is the same as you get while masturbating. After all, as Woody Allen said, "masturbating is having sex with someone I love," but there is no doubt that emotions implicit in the sexual act enrich the physical sensations and bring it to other levels that are really hard to describe.

In this chapter I am going to talk about sex with your partner. Whether steady or unstable, serious or casual, the relationship established when two people make love is perhaps the most intimate and personal that humans can enjoy. You may have been told that when you truly love someone, failure to reach an orgasm while making love with him is not that important. Maybe you have been told that the feeling of intimacy is so great, the tenderness so crucial, and the communication between the two so intense that an orgasm becomes secondary. Sorry, but I disagree. If it only happens very rarely, maybe it has no bearing, but to never reach it is something certainly frustrating. As my friend Natalia puts it: "Not getting to orgasm while making love with my partner pains me. Sex without an orgasm is like kissing your mother on the forehead: tender, intimate, warm, but...clearly insufficient."

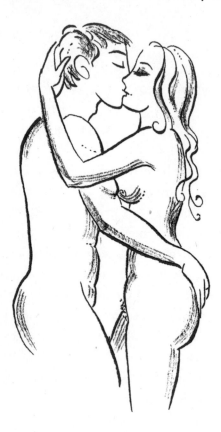

Your body, your mind, your whole being needs to orgasm while making love to feel satisfied, complete, content, and relaxed. Of course, this is not about your obsessing over an orgasm so much that you are unable to enjoy every moment that the sexual relationship with someone offers you. Rather, it is the opposite: to have an orgasm easily during sex, you should be fully relaxed, surrendered, and able to enjoy every one of the small and minimal details of the relationship with your partner. Do not worry. Relax and keep reading, because I will show you what to do to make sex with your partner get to where it needs to get: the ecstasy of you both. And if that should occur at the same time, even better. Shared pleasure is the best way to enjoy sex and feel an intense orgasm.

"I like to climb on top of my boyfriend—play with him, put my breasts in his mouth; I move up and down and rub my pelvis against his thighs and his belly. When I suddenly put his penis in my vagina, he literally goes crazy."

Adriana, 37 years old

As far as sex is concerned, one of the most widespread ideas is that a man can have an orgasm in just 3 minutes, while women need between 20 minutes and half an hour to get there. This is absolutely false. A woman who regularly masturbates and has reached an adequate control of her vaginal muscles can have an orgasm in just 3 minutes with the proper clitoral stimulation. So, imagine the possibilities that this offers you when making love with your partner. You have already learned in the previous chapter how you can reach an orgasm easily. Now do not hesitate to put it to use when you have company.

"My boyfriend told me once that he masturbated before making love to me so that he could then take longer to have an orgasm. I also masturbate, but for just the opposite reason: before an orgasm, I touch myself until I feel a huge level of excitement...but I stop right before it. So, when we make love, I practically orgasm when I want."

Esmeralda, 30 years old

There are several ways in which you can control your orgasm, so that when you make love with your partner, you get to control when you want to get there, and even do it at the same time with him.

One of them is expressed in Esmeralda's testimony that you just read. That way, you reach such a high degree of excitement before intercourse that when the time comes, you can trigger an orgasm with a few wisely directed movements. Another is masturbating during sex. In the position best suited for your physical needs, we will now offer you a guide to the more convenient positions; your partner's own movement will stimulate your clitoris directly, and that will be enough. But if that is not the case, you can resort to masturbating. At first you may think that your partner will find it strange, but you may be surprised when he finds it exciting to feel how you masturbate and see you become even more aroused as he moves inside you.

In any case, it is always important that you take calm pleasure during foreplay. Kisses and caresses stimulate your sexual desire and put your sexual organs in the best position to complete their mission and make you enjoy it the most.

I ALSO KNOW HOW TO FAKE IT

No woman likes to think that her partner is not enjoying making love. If you have seen a pornographic movie, you have seen the participants sighing and gesturing as if they were effusively enjoying it the whole time: they are good actresses. In fact, they are likely thinking about the fact that the next day they have to take their child to the doctor, or whether what they will get for the movie will pay off the car. In real life, pretending is never a good way to actually reach an orgasm. I must admit that I also faked it a lot, until I discovered that what I really wanted in a sexual relationship was enjoyment. Not that my partner should think that I was enjoying it, but I should actually enjoy it. Everything changed in my relationships ever since.

A relationship in which I get no sexual pleasure is not worth it. Now I know how to orgasm regardless of whether my partner is an expert or novice, or knows the points I find pleasurable...because I learned how to tell him.

It is said that there are no frigid women, just inexperienced men. That is one of the most sexist statements I have ever heard in my life. In any case, there will be inexperienced or ignorant women, or, at least, women who do not know their own sexuality. When you know what you like, when you know your body and know how it reacts, when you are sure of where and how you like to be touched to get pleasure, all you have to do is guide your partner, or do it yourself.

Communication is essential for him to know how to make you quiver. And if he disagrees, or does not like to be led, or thinks he is so "manly" that his erection is all you need to orgasm, he is probably not someone worth your while, and you should make it clear to him that either he changes or he'd better find someone else who is willing to put up with his arrogance.

THE 10 MOST EXCITING POSITIONS

Much is heard or seen in magazines or movies about positions. Some seem more appropriate for a circus than for a sexual encounter between two people of different genders. There are many positions for making love. One is no better than the others. It just depends on the individuals, the situation, and the environment. It is not the same thing to make love in an elevator with a stranger before arriving at your floor as it is to do it in the suite of a luxury hotel on your wedding night after three bottles of champagne. That is why it is important to have all possible information regarding the most desirable positions, and that you chose them at any given time, for yourself, your partner, and whatever it is you want. Sometimes what you want is a quick orgasm because you have to go to work and do not want to be late; other times you have all afternoon or the entire night to take chances and try a few things.

1. **The missionary position.** Also called "Adam and Eve" or "marriage." It is the most common position in the Mediterranean area. In it, the man lies on top of the woman, facing her. The woman can wrap her legs around the man's

body or just spread her legs open. If you are the type who has her clitoris connected to the labia of the vagina, your partner's pelvic motion will be enough to indirectly stimulate you and provoke a very intense orgasm. If not, your partner can stimulate your clitoris with his pelvic bone; the penetration angle will be slightly different, but the end result will be just as good.

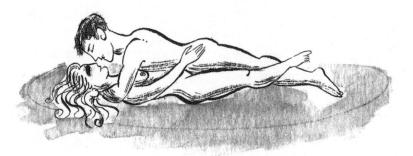

Ideally, the man will keep a pace of a few thrusts, four or five, then briefly stop, and then continue with the same pace. It is also very pleasant for the man to make a circle with his movements, so as to not only push and pull but keep constant pressure on the pubic area and the woman's clitoris. Ideally, it is up to you to guide the speed and pressure of the movement. You can do it with your hands or his buttocks.... They are so erotic!

"Although a little tarnished, it is the position that my boyfriend and I prefer. We look into each other's eyes; we can kiss with tenderness and passion and see how pleasure takes a hold of us. There is complete bodily contact, and the feeling of fullness is unmatched. We like it so much that we have to make an effort to try other positions."

Amanda, 31 years old

2. **Woman on top.** This is ideal if you want to take the initiative. You can control the depth of penetration and the pace of your movements. It also allows both you and your partner to have easy access to the clitoris with your hands. If your boyfriend is also particularly soft and gentle when he caresses your breasts, this may be your ideal position.

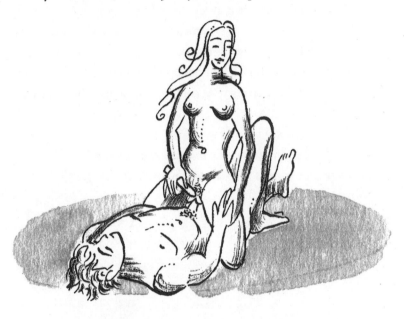

If you like to have your G-spot stimulated, you can sit on his penis, so that when you move, you will stimulate the anterior vaginal wall, and I assure you that you will have a very, very good time. Just keep in mind not to land on him with all of your weight!

"I love it when Susi and I make love with her on top of me. I can see her entire body, caress her breasts, see and touch her vagina and clitoris. But what I like best of all is to see the passion reflected in her face."

Agustín, 25 years old

3. **Woman on top, facing away.** A very attractive variant of the earlier stance is for you to face away from your partner. You have access to the clitoris, and your partner can stimulate and caress your anus and buttocks. Having no eye contact, you can fantasize as much as you feel like and make all the gestures you want. Sometimes it is pleasantly liberating to look fierce, without any fear of what your face may look like! In this position, you are the one who controls the movements, but you have to do it carefully, because until you get a good rhythm, it is not difficult for the penis to slip out. If you hold on to his feet as you move in a gentle swaying motion, you can get him to delay his orgasm.

"I like this position because the movements are smooth and harmonious. More than going in and out of my vagina, his penis is always inside me while we touch forcefully and gently backwards and forwards. Wow!"

Adela, 39 years old

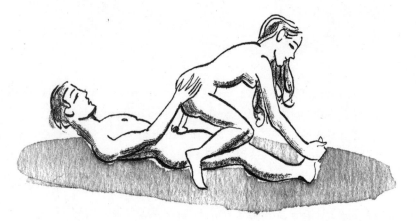

4. **Facing spoons.** This position will be very comfortable. Lying on your sides, facing each other, neither has to support the weight of the other. The penetration can be very deep. With a

smooth gentleness and a good coupling of the legs, the whole genital area is directly and intensely stimulated. Also notice that in this position, your partner can control his movements well and prolong his orgasm.

"Lying on my side next to Miguel, and feeling as he penetrates me slowly as he opens my vagina with his leg is the most delicious thing I know."

Andrea, 26 years old

5. **Spooning.** If you are pregnant, this position is for you. Lie down on your side, just as your partner lies on his side and enters you from behind. There is no position more comfortable than this one. You can prolong intercourse for as long as you please without getting tired. Both he and you have easy access to the clitoris if you so desire. It is so nice for him to hug you from behind and caress your breasts while moving inside you as the feeling of pleasure increases slowly! If you open and lift your knees a little, penetration becomes easier and deeper. And if you really want him to go deep, bend your waist forward: the position becomes a bit more "wild," but you can have your moments!

Another variant of this position is to sit on his thighs backward with knees bent. Penetration like this is very nice because he can stimulate your clitoris or caress your breasts while you set the pace.

"We discovered this position when I was pregnant, but then we continued practicing it with increasing frequency. We start slowly, but as we get into it, sometimes the bed begins to bump against the wall, and it is as though the patter is going at our own pace, and... Wow!"

Emma, 40 years old

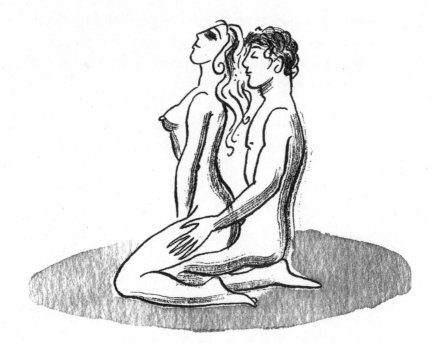

6. **The cat.** Bored? You no longer know what to do to break the monotony of sex with your partner? Try this: with him standing, holding you in his arms, wrap your legs around his hips. You might think that this looks uncomfortable, but I assure you that the penetration is very deep, and his pelvis presses so hard against your clitoris, that your orgasm will not delay, just as you rub up against each other. If you do not have much time, or if you are in an elevator or in the office's broom closet and there is no room for much else, this position is perfect.

To make it a more comfortable position, you can rest your buttocks on the edge of a table or a tall stool.

"Making love in the kitchen is the most exciting experience I've ever had. There I am making sandwiches, and suddenly here comes Juan, and he starts to caress me passionately, he lifts my skirt, pushing me until my buttocks bump against the edge of the table, and we go for it! I feel that his penis is huge and my clitoris is about to explode. It's delicious!"

Amina, 41 years old

7. **The cart.** You lie down on your back. He drops to his knees and, looking passionately into your eyes, holds you by your hips. You raise your waist upward so that your sexual organs come into contact. He has your vagina in front of him and can no longer contain his excitement. Your labia swell and open. Your open legs stretch your genital muscles. Can you imagine it? Penetration is not that easy, but when you get it, you will have the most intense orgasm of your life.

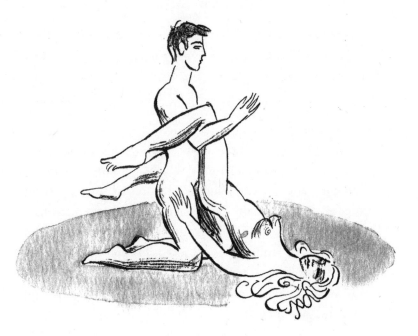

"I saw this pose in a porn movie and found it very uncomfortable and difficult. But when I met Julian at night, I could not resist and asked him that we try it. I've never seen him so passionate. I've never enjoyed it as much."

Cecilia, 23 years old

8. **The doggy.** This is a very, very exciting position. At the outset, it may seem a little erotic, but if you are passionate, or have a steady relationship with the same person, this position will open doors to new sensations. This is you with your knees, hands, or elbows on the floor, the carpet, or the mattress. The man, also kneeling, enters you from behind. The penetration is very shallow, and the angle can be easily varied. In this position, the penis vigorously stimulates the anterior vaginal wall where the G-spot is located, so that orgasms can become really intense and delicious.

"Making love is fine. It is nice and pleasant, but sometimes I'm so excited that I feel like doing something stronger, something like fucking. The puppy is an ideal position for these occasions."

Alicia, 25 years old

9. **The scissors.** In this position, your legs and his are intertwined like scissors. It has all the variations you can imagine, and it always allows a perfect fit for your sexual organs. It is especially recommended when the man has a small penis, because the two organs meet easily, and thus the feeling of "fullness" is achieved through the perfect fit, regardless of the size of the penis. Moreover, the man's pelvis can easily stimulate your clitoris, so that the orgasm is fast and guaranteed.

"Feeling contact with his thighs clenched tightly against mine is what I like so much. And the pressure on my clitoris is so constant and so sweet! We have no problems pacing our movements, and we can caress and kiss each other at will. It is certainly my favorite position."

Iris, 38 years old

10. **Dangerous summits.** You stand facing away from your partner. Then you bend at the waist and support yourself on your hands or your knees, or on a chair or the sink. You raise your leg a little so that he, who is also standing, can enter you from behind. Once he has penetrated you, bring your legs together tightly to squeeze his penis really hard. It is a perfect position for a quick rendezvous, because he does not even need to take off his pants. We do not always have all the time in the world! With one of your hands, you can stimulate your clitoris and speed up your orgasm.

"When Manuel put me in this position, it seemed a little dirty, too unromantic. Of course I did not know what I was getting myself into. Do you know how exciting it is to do it in a nightclub's restroom, for example? I think that since then I love him even more."

Berta, 24 years old

Helpful tips

When it comes to sex, believe me when I say that everything should be permitted. Whether you are enjoying it alone or in company, why put any limits to the imagination? Consider that, according to the Kama Sutra, there are over 500 positions for making love. I have only covered the ten that seem the most exciting, but the truth is that there is no limit other than that which you impose on yourself. Yet this is nothing extraordinary, bizarre, or weird. There are simple little things, objects, common things in any household, which can lead to a lot of play in increasing sexual arousal and pleasure. We suggest some, and we invite you to complete the list yourself:

A mirror. Placed on the ceiling or the wall, it can act as a powerful aphrodisiac.

A high stool. The type seen at bar counters. When used to support your buttocks in the cat pose, or to rest your hands on during "dangerous summits," it will add a special touch to your relationships.

A wide bed with a hard mattress. When you are kneeling or standing up, it will help you go into all kinds of variations in the positions that we have explained.

A pillow. It seems incredible! A simple pillow under your buttocks when you are in the missionary position, for example, can facilitate contact between your partner's pelvis and your clitoris...and you already know what that means.

Warm water. Just like that! How about in the bathtub?

Lights, colors, and sounds. All senses play an important role in arousal and pleasure. Soft lighting, nice colors—always with something red to increase the passion—appropriate music...it will help you prepare the ideal scenario.... So, what are you waiting for?

Fantasies and orgasms are inseparable

In a previous chapter, you learned that sex starts in the mind. Sexual fantasies are essential for strong, deep, and delicious orgasms. Once again, do not impose limits on your imagination...better yet, never limit yourself. Pleasure does not depend only on your anatomy. Concentrating on what you are doing is absolutely essential. Fantasies will help you get there.

"I loved Juan very much, but I had no other choice than to acknowledge that he was not a particularly exciting guy. One day, I imagined a couple of friends making love while Juan watched them. After a while, Juan was included in the game and joined them in a ménage à trois. I got so excited that I had a very intense orgasm almost immediately. I've never had an experience like that in real life, and the truth is that I am not interested in having it, but by playing with my imagination, Juan became for me an absolutely irresistible man."

Susana, 33 years old

Having sexual fantasies is completely normal. You should not be scared by that, even if the content is a little strong. The fact that you get excited when thinking of a man forcing you to do something in particular does not mean that you would like for that to happen in reality. In your imagination there is no pain. It is a manifestation of your creativity and an invaluable aid to realizing your desires. I am not sure why, but throughout my experience, I have been able to prove that in this regard, men have a great advantage over us. The women with whom I have spoken are generally limited in their fantasies to making love with their partner, but men…you cannot even begin to imagine where they are able to go in their imagination to get excited! This is probably due to the guilt with which women have regarded sexuality for generations, even when it is only in fantasies. But those days are over.

We live in a world where the right to think whatever you want and letting your imagination run wildly without any limits is fully accepted. Enough with the guilt and the false inhibitions. Do not forget that, by nature, all that is forbidden attracts us. Let your mind wander all the way to the top!

A very high percentage of women (over 90%) need sexual fantasies in order to reach an orgasm while masturbating, and a considerable number (over 70%) have them while making love with their partners. Does this mean that we should fantasize about our partners while making love? Not necessarily! If you find it more exciting to imagine your upstairs neighbor or George Clooney, or both, naked and whispering stimulating things in your ear, why not allow yourself?

Imagination is harmless. It is simply about helping yourself focus on sex and unplugging from your daily routine, with all your energy, because in doing so, you will enjoy your sexual experience much more, and you will have an orgasm more easily.

I DO NOT KNOW HOW TO FANTASIZE

That is not true. Everyone knows how to fantasize. What could be happening is that you are afraid, or you are under the impression that you are doing something wrong or at least inappropriate. I know many women who feel guilty because they have sexual fantasies about their husband's friends, or movie stars or singers. This makes no sense. Fantasy is absolutely free and does not hurt anyone. A woman is no more faithful or more decent because she only has erotic fantasies about her partner. Faithfulness and decency are elsewhere. Fantasizing about different men is absolutely normal, and you should not try to stop it. In fact, the appeal of having sexual fantasies is that they leave us free to have any sexual experience outside of reality. Enjoy this great advantage! How about a passionate romance with Brad Pitt while you shower? Having certain fantasies does not mean that you truly want them to become reality. Consider them more like a game, or assistance, something important to help you focus on sex and enjoy it.

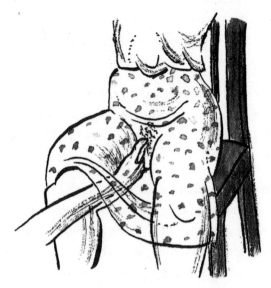

"Do I have fantasies? Many and of every kind. I have fantasies about my gynecologist, where I imagine him penetrating me on the examining table, with two men holding me down at the same time; one is inside my vagina and another in my anus. I imagine myself making love with someone while my partner watches us, or that a stranger fondles me under the table at a restaurant. Normally, I do not have time to come up with an elaborate fantasy while I am making love because I orgasm quickly, but it helps me a lot to bring to mind quick images like those I just mentioned."

Isabel, 39 years old

HOW DO I DO IT?

Nevertheless, if you are the type of person who considers herself incapable of fantasizing in a pleasant and fun way, follow these tips:

1. **Discard the stories that have a beginning, a middle, and an end.** We agreed that fantasy is free. Forget the plot! Focus on particular details and brief images that you find exciting: a glance, a touch, penetration, kissing.

2. **Images need not be sexually explicit.** Sometimes it is more exciting when it is romantic and sensual, like an unexpected touch, or a tight embrace at the end of a cliff, as the sun sets at sea.

3. **In almost every fantasy** the most exciting parts are often the small details: imagining the face of an attractive man at the moment you orgasm; a passionate encounter in an unexpected situation, like in the dining room at home or in the backseat of the car; a certain special touch that "turns you on."

4. Practice all kinds of fantasies while masturbating; you will see how it helps when you do it with your partner.

Now that you have read my tips, lie down on the couch, turn off the TV, and turn on soft lighting. Unplug the phone, and if you can, turn off the doorbell. A little soft music can also come in handy. Start exploring your body slowly while your mind finds exciting situations. You can start in a small and intimate restaurant. A stranger that you have been looking at for a while, because you find him attractive, gets up from his table and appears to be approaching you. The next image you see can be a passionate kiss with that stranger at the restaurant's exit or in the car...and now you can go on your own! Imagine that hot men caress you, or watch you touching yourself and come up to you and fondle you. Remember that in your imagination everything is allowed! You would be surprised by the high percentage of women who get excited at the thought of being forced by a man or several men; if that is the case, do not deprive yourself! Give yourself permission, let yourself go...and keep touching yourself as you do so. Remember what I told you in the section on masturbation. If you feel like you are going to have an orgasm, stop for a moment and continue imagining; the next wave of excitement will be even stronger. Go back to the previous situation, or change it if you no longer find it as exciting; let your mind wander freely to places and situations that really prove irresistible to you. Think about your favorite actor, or the upstairs neighbor, or your friend's husband...anything goes; this is nothing more than just a fantasy! Imagine how he approaches you, smiles at you, and begins to caress you. When you feel the excitement rise up again, and it starts to become an orgasm, arch your hips, moan, or say the words that come to you and that will increase your arousal. You might even feel like screaming. The interesting thing is that your thoughts will rise in tone and intensity as your arousal grows, until you reach an orgasm in your fantasy...and in reality.

Another possible way to start a fantasy can be the memory of a previous sexual experience that proved to be enjoyable. It is not about imagining it exactly the same way it was. The secret is in reimagining it with all kinds of details that may not have happened but that are right now most tempting to you. He is now even sweeter and gentler than on that occasion, the light is dimmer, and the position is even more exciting. You could even try writing your favorite fantasy and describing every detail. Do not worry if you do not get a script worthy of Pedro Almodóvar. It does not matter if the scenes do not have a credible continuity. This is about you putting down in writing the details, situations, and caresses that excite you. You can also include the words you like to hear when making love. Then, later, when you go to put your imagination into practice again, read what you have written, and that can really help you begin to imagine.

SHOULD I SHARE MY FANTASIES WITH MY PARTNER?

Relationships are very personal, and even more so when sex is involved. There is no single and final answer to that question. It depends on the type of relationship you have with your partner. It depends on your personality and his. What should be clear is that you are not obligated to share your fantasies. We all have a private world that we do not share with anyone. Imagination is an essential part of that privacy. Perhaps it is the only territory in which we are truly free. There is no need to explain or say why we imagine something. We do it simply because we like it, because we enjoy it, and because it excites us. Respecting that privacy is essential in a relationship. If sharing these fantasies with your partner will help improve your relationship, do it. But if you feel that he will not understand you, or it embarrasses you a little, or you believe that this is something that only belongs to you, do not worry at all. Nobody has the right to invade that part of you.

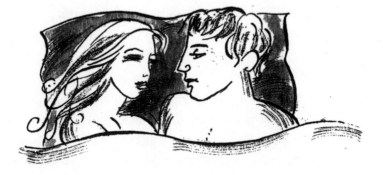

If your partner gets irritated and asks you again what you are wondering while you make love, just tell him what you know he would like to hear. You can say that you only think of him, and that it excites you to think of what you do in real life, or that he is such a good lover that you are unable to imagine anything else, because he excites you so much that your imagination gets blocked. Anything to make him feel happy. Do not think that you are lying. In any case, it would be his fault for trying to invade a territory that does not belong to him.

But it can also be another type of situation. Maybe your partner is so open and understanding to hearing your fantasies that he not only does not mind it, but it excites him even more. If that is the case, go ahead. As my 35-year-old friend Adela told me, "I never imagined that I could tell my sex dreams to a man so frankly. With my previous partner that was unthinkable. So I knew right away that Fernando was the man of my life; I tell him everything I imagine, and not only does he not get angry, but he gets even more excited and loves me with more passion." I must admit that Adela's situation is much like the ideal that we all crave—a completely frank and open relationship where you share absolutely everything. But based on my experience with men, do not open up too much on this topic, because men are usually very sensitive and tend to feel hurt if you tell them that you had an almost unbearable orgasm imagining that you had a romance on the beach with your favorite movie star.

TOYS AND STIMULI

Humans are the only animals that use fantasy to have an orgasm. We do not need the visual stimulus for sexual satisfaction because the mind is so powerful that it can replace it. However, there are many external aids that enhance the imagination and, in some cases, cause or increase pleasure.

In this section I will offer a wide variety of things that you can use alone or with your partner, for your own arousal, to help you fantasize, or to provoke an orgasm. We will start talking about "toys" that can be found in specialty stores.

Ben Wa balls. These are two metal balls joined by a latex string. They are inserted into the vagina and move every time that the pelvis moves, causing a peculiar excitement and, in some cases, an orgasm. They can be worn in any situation—be careful, because in a business meeting, your gestures of pleasure can give you away! They are recommended for women who have underdeveloped vaginal muscles, because their movement helps strengthen them. Many times, they are hollow with a smaller ball inside that hits the walls of the big one when it moves and cause even more excitement.

Vibrators. They come in all colors, shapes, and even flavors. They run on disposable batteries or a battery that is charged with a plug. If you have never had an orgasm while masturbating, run to buy one at the first sex shop you find! Start by using it directly on the clitoris, and get ready, because those sensations are indescribable. You can also use vibrators with your partner and apply them on different parts of your body.

Penis extenders. They are so called because they are like a condom with a tip that has a sort of ridge that gives the feeling of penis enlargement. With that little bump, your partner's penis has easy access to the G-spot. Longer or shorter, you will never forget the feeling that it will give you.

COCK RINGS

Does your partner suffer from premature ejaculation? These metal rings are placed on the penis and testicles, and he gets a longer-lasting erection. Encourage him to give them a try! You will enjoy it more, and it will make him feel better.

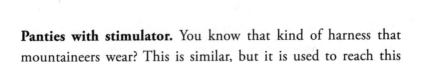

Panties with stimulator. You know that kind of harness that mountaineers wear? This is similar, but it is used to reach this other type of climax. Place these panties below your normal panties; where they meet your vagina, there is a small protrusion that rubs the clitoris. Can you imagine wearing them while you stroll through the park?

Massage gloves. Yes, like the ones you wear in the snow, but in latex...and they vibrate! You can use them for your morning shower, use them to caress yourself, or give them to your partner to touch you wherever you like.

Condoms. They may not be an instrument of pleasure, but for many reasons, it is very advisable to use them in relationships with a partner. They come in all shapes, colors, and flavors imaginable. How about a bit of raspberry-flavored oral sex?

Suction pumps. They run on disposable batteries, or a battery that is charged by the electrical current, just as a mobile phone is. They are placed over the vagina or clitoris, and you can imagine their effect!

So much for the "toys." Let us talk now about other external "aids." Are you still unable to fantasize? Do you still find it difficult to imagine your favorite actor embracing you in his arms or giving you oral pleasure? You just have to keep reading more.

Erotic literature. Does that not sound much better than porn? In our world the "politically correct" is increasingly important. However, do not be afraid to call things by their proper names. To make this easier, and provide a resource that you can use in conversation, we will differentiate erotica from porn. Not that one is better than the other; it is simply that each one has its role and different effects depending on the person.

Maybe you are one of those women who find romantic stories exciting—especially if they also contain some explicit sex, more or less. There are plenty of novels that meet those requirements. I will give just a few titles that you may find interesting: *Lady Chatterley's Lover* by D. H. Lawrence and *The Diary of Anaïs Nin* and *The Ages of Lulu* by Almudena Grandes. They are not specifically sexual stories, but they do contain a lot of sex, which may suggest many starting points for your future fantasies. For a lot of women, the way in which sex acts are described in these stories are more exciting than explicit sex scenes in a movie.

Another interesting aspect of what we might call "erotica" can be found in women's magazines. Photos and stories of naked couples making love can be suggestive, but they are nothing compared to the actual testimonials that are published in many magazines. Reading about others' sexual experiences is something irresistible. You may be surprised to discover how exciting it is to know other people's intimate details.

Pornography. Have you always heard that pornography is for men? For women, seeing how many partners are exchanged continuously, while having oral sex or masturbating at the same time, is something they find unpleasant...or at least, so they say. Have you really tried watching a pornographic movie on an early Saturday morning? Men do it without shame. They even gather in bars to see it while bursting into laughter from excitement...and from impotence. We are more refined, more sensitive, and we do not like to express our desires in such a vile way. But that does not mean that we do not get aroused! The visual stimulus is perhaps most powerful when it comes to increasing excitement, and with it the achievement of an orgasm, so why not try it? Forget any prejudices. Do not think of it as a "guy thing." I assure you that if you relax and put yourself in front of the screen with a willing mind, your engine will get going in no time, and you will not be able to avoid touching yourself until you have an orgasm. They do it, so why shouldn't we?

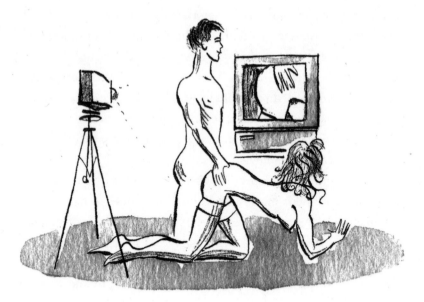

If your partner agrees, you can try making love while watching a pornographic film. Does that seem too bold for you? For most men, even if they say otherwise, a daring woman is irresistible. Can you imagine the amount of possibilities that will open up to you both? You could even make your own porn. It is not about recording it in a video, but to act as if you were doing so. Place the video camera so that it focuses on the bed, and have the television in front so that you can watch it. Light up the scene properly and begin to act as if you were in one of those movies. You could be lying there, acting as if you do not want anything. He comes into the room. You did not expect him, but it gives you a lot of joy to see him, and you show it by giving him a hug and a kiss. Then you go on to better things, and he will start to slowly undress you. The camera records it, and you watch it on the screen... I leave the rest up to you, but I assure you that Sharon Stone would pale with envy.

TASTE

The mouth is an orifice that serves as an inlet and outlet for our bodies. Through it we bring in food, liquid, and pleasure. If you close your eyes and go over your body, not to mention the genitals, with vanilla ice cream, or some peach jam, for example, your partner's exploration of your body with his tongue will be much more exciting and will bring you closer to having an orgasm.

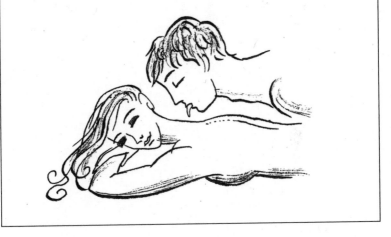

Sounds. All senses play a role in sexual arousal and pleasure. I remember a song that I heard often when I was a teenager. It was called *Je t'aime, moi non plus,* and in the background I could hear the moans of a couple making love until they had an orgasm. Every time I heard it at a party, I had to run to the bathroom! Get a recording in which you hear something similar. And if that is not easy for you to get, set up a recorder the next time you make love with your partner or you have an orgasm by yourself. Keep it in a safe place, because if you are bored one afternoon and you do not get aroused, just relax a little and start playing the recording. Its effects are powerful!

Guys, this is what we like!

This chapter is for the guys. They are so convinced of their skills! They talk about their "exploits" like supermen. And yet they can be so wrong sometimes! They touch our breasts as if they were squeezing lemons, or tighten them so much that we are almost unable to breathe. Let us give them a hand. We are going to tell our secrets, what we like to do, and how we like to do it. Of course, we are not all the same, and some of us like some things more than others, but I am sure that all women would support the tips I am going to give here. It is all so simple in the end!

SOME MISCONCEPTIONS

Men, when you get together in a pub, there are two topics of conversation: football and women. If an alien looked in on your gatherings, he would think that you know everything about what we like and why we are attracted to you...unless the alien was a woman. It is difficult to conceive of such an accumulation of nonsense. Almost everything in those coffee chats in which you express what we like as women is as close to reality as Tampa Bay is to the North Pole. Luckily, in the end, you are much more sensitive than you would seem to be when you are with friends, and when you make the effort, you know the proper way to treat us.

Anyway, let us take a look at some of these "theories" that are often heard in discussions between men and that have as much to do with reality as chalk does with cheese.

The clitoris is the most sensitive part of a woman. "A man has sex to feel good; a woman has to feel good to have sex." Do you understand the difference? If you think that a couple of kisses and a few squeezes of her breasts, and everything is ready for penetration and for you to hit her clitoris like a golf ball, you are wrong. For a woman to have a fulfilling sexual relationship, to reach an orgasm easily, she has to feel desired, meaning sexually attractive. That is the first key; it is the most sensitive point: sex starts in the mind, as we have seen. The first requirement for a woman to consider you to be an attractive man and want to make love to you is that you find her attractive, and that you be able to make her feel that. You will be surprised to know that if a woman does not feel sexy, she will never reach an orgasm, no matter how you grip her clitoris.

Women have to be dominated from the start. It is not a bad idea if you intend to build a house by starting from the roof. But if you insist on that, it is quite likely that you will have a difficult time getting sex for free. Women want to be treated as equals in a sexual relationship. Sometimes it is nice to feel dominated... but sometimes it is not. It is much more important to be able to convey to a woman the assurance that you do not consider her to be inferior in any way, by any demonstration of "manliness" you can imagine. If you get her to feel treated as an equal, and you know how to create the right situation, it is likely that she will find it pleasant and enjoyable to "feel dominated." But do not forget that roles change sometimes, and that she may feel at any a given moment as though she were a "man-eater" who can "dominate" anyone who crosses her path.

WOMEN LIKE US TO GET "STRAIGHT TO THE POINT"

If there is something that a woman hates, it is for you to go "straight to the point." Give her time. Play with her. Allow her to enter into the situation completely. The "preparations" are essential for any woman. The more time you devote to her, the more pleasant the culmination will be. Do not forget that a woman needs to be lubricated enough to welcome penetration with pleasure. If you obsess over penetrating her as quickly as possible, all you will get is...for her to close her legs and send you away. A very erotic and exciting game consists of mutually feeding each other aphrodisiac delicacies (like oysters, asparagus, etc.) in the style of the movie *9 ½ WEEKS*.

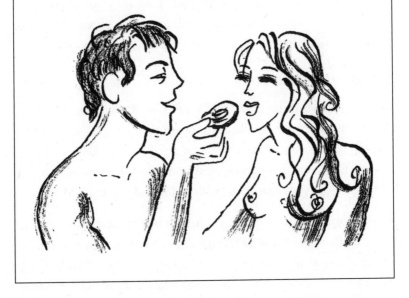

The size of the penis is very important. This is as important as whether your neighbor is named Maria or Federica! The most sensitive part of a woman's vagina is in the muscles around it and the G-spot. And the G-spot is less than an inch inside the vagina! Do you know a friend whose erect penis is no longer than two inches? Well, there is no need for more! In fact, too large a penis can touch the cervix and cause pain. The feeling of "fullness" that you think a large penis provides is achieved with a suitable position. Check out the chapter on positions!

Women like "violent" sex. You have seen too many movies! In real life, things rarely happen the same way as on the screen. A deep, intense, long-lasting orgasm, even the case of multiple orgasms, gets much better with rhythmic, long, smooth thrusts. If at any time your partner wants a little more "violence," let her be the one to suggest it. Do not be inept! If you are paying attention, you will fully realize when she wants you to accelerate or squeeze a little more. But if you only go by what you think she likes, chances are that you will finish so fast that she will not get to tell the difference between making love to you and you tripping on the doorway.

Some helpful tips

Pay attention, because now I will speak not of what you think, but of what we women really like. This opens up a great opportunity for you. If you know how to take advantage of it, it is likely that, from now on, you may have more pleasurable sexual relationships...and may finally get your partner to really enjoy making love with you.

Undress me gently. Stripping clothes off is very exciting in a movie, but actually this is not something we like, nor does it turn us on. We prefer to enjoy an exciting preamble. Hugs, caresses, kisses, slowly discovering the body...that is the secret! Make her feel that her naked-ness excites you, that every bit of her body that you discover increases your desire, that you find appealing every inch of skin where you get rid of her clothing. Make her feel it...and tell her so! Softly, in her ear, between kisses, caresses, and cuddles. That will again make her feel attractive and desired, and increase her confidence and sense of security and relaxation. A woman who is not relaxed cannot reach an orgasm, and it is hard to relax if you tear off her clothes and throw yourself on top of her like a sack of potatoes. Help her feel confident. Remember: "A woman has to feel good to have sex." Only in this way will she get to a quick and pleasurable orgasm.

Kiss me a lot. If you want to be a passionate lover and excite your partner from the beginning, you will have to make an effort when it comes to kissing. Be imaginative when you kiss, concentrate on the contact between the lips, and try to synchronize the movement of your tongues for a complete blending of the two. Kisses act as soothing balm in the beginning, filling us with security and confidence, and as a starter toward pleasure, as their intensity grows. Start kissing only the corners of your partner's mouth; they are highly erogenous. Then offer her the soft and inviting inside of your lips in a deep, intimate, and erotic kiss. While you kiss, caress her hair and neck. Run your tongue over her gums and the edge of her tongue. When you have done all that, nibble her lips gently. Stop in the middle of a deep kiss and sigh without pulling away from her mouth so that she can feel the warmth of your breath. You can take advantage of this break to tell her how attractive and desirable she is to you.

I AM ATTRACTIVE AND DESIRABLE

We like to have our clitoris caressed...but not in the first minute. You have already learned that sex begins in the mind. Prove to your partner that she is the sexiest and most desirable woman. Kiss her often. Call her at work to tell her that you love her. Give her flowers for no special reason. Embrace her tenderly when you get home...even if you are tired. Tell her that she seems slimmer and more attractive. It is the best way to get her to orgasm. Don Juan did not seduce women because he had a very big penis. He was irresistible to them because he made them feel unique and desirable, because he knew how to interpret their desires and how to get closer to what they wanted, because he wrote them beautiful love letters and he continually praised their beauty. They surrendered to him almost beforehand. They felt attractive, desirable, and unique. They went to bed with him...and enjoyed intense orgasms. Because, usually, a man who can treat women like this will also know which steps to follow in any sexual relationship and how to play up his lover's sensitive points in the most appropriate way. If you keep reading, you will find some practical tips in this regard as well.

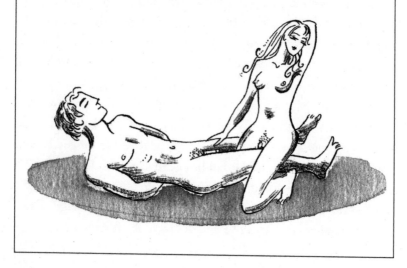

Take your time. A good technique is to increase tenfold the time you think is needed for your girl to be suitably aroused. Four hugs and two badly given kisses do not count. A woman's body needs time, trust, and relaxation to be sensitive to the touch. The vagina has to change in size, it has to open, and it needs to be properly lubricated. The clitoris has to become erect, just like your penis, and it takes a while to get there. Before any penetration, stop at every part of the woman's body. At the mouth and face, breasts and belly, thighs and hips. Caress each of these parts with softness, sweetness, and passion. Kiss her in every corner; penetration should only occur when both of you are desperate for it to happen. This will speed up your orgasm...and hers. If you do it this way, the orgasms will be so intense and deep that you will notice how the neighbors look at you with more respect in the elevator in the morning.

Interpret her answers. If you hear that she starts moaning, continue what you are doing and do not move on quickly to something else. Always follow the suggestions made to you, whether by word—unusual—or hand gestures and indications. When you feel her lift up her thighs or she squeezes your head against her with more intensity, it means that she wants more pressure. If her hands clench your buttocks with fast and insistent movements, it means that she wants to speed it up. And when you feel her breathing stop and her body tense, she is starting to have an orgasm...or she heard the baby cry in the room next door.

Say something. We like to hear how you enjoy it. But not only through groans. Do not be afraid to speak. Tell your partner how good you feel. Tell her how much pleasure you feel in what you are doing. With details. You cannot imagine how exciting it is for a woman to hear from the lips of a man who is enjoying himself like crazy that he cannot hold it in any longer—to hear from a man who is in heaven that if pleasure keeps increasing, he is going to die. Many times, women orgasm sooner because we hear things like this from our partner rather than from having our G-spot touched.

THE APPROPRIATE SEQUENCE

Imagine that you are already in bed. You have undressed your partner with all the softness and care that I advised you about a little earlier. Now I am going to propose a sequence, a timing, for her to have an unforgettable sexual experience. If you follow my advice, tomorrow morning when you look at yourself in the mirror to shave, you are going to sing with more self-assurance than Ricky Martin.

Caresses and kisses, caresses and kisses. Lie down next to her. Caress her hair. Gently, tenderly. Kiss her forehead and eyebrows. Many times. With soft, tender kisses, with very little pressure and soft, delicate, continuous contact. One of your hands can go slowly down the side of her face, the back of her ears, her neck, and, very delicately, around her breasts. Kiss her on the mouth, half opening her lips a little, as if "sinking" your lips into hers. Let her be the first to use her tongue. If she does it, follow her, rub it gently with yours, and insert it into her mouth a little. Do not go all the way into the back of her mouth, or you will make her feel nausea and break the charm.

Concentrate now on her ears. Do not insert your tongue—we do not like to have our ears sucked! Rather, kiss the back of her ears softly and repeatedly. Caress the lobe with your tongue. In front and behind. Gently.

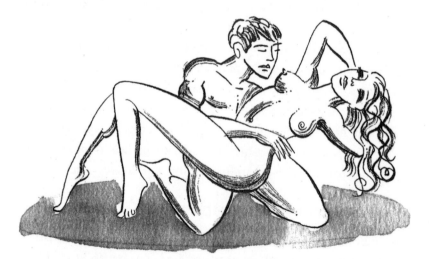

Make your way toward her breasts. Not roughly! The breasts are extremely sensitive. Caress both at once, from top to bottom and with little circular motions without touching the nipples...yet.

Begin to gently lick her breast in a circular manner and from the periphery to the center. Go with your tongue to the areola and stop there a few moments. Do you hear her moaning? Then continue with the same for a while. Then go on to the nipple. Always in circles and gently. Try pressing a little and feel her reaction. It is important to know how to interpret her answers: if she caresses the back of your head, press a little more. You will notice that her nipples will harden. Suck them gently. She will let you know how far you should push.

Then, always slowly and gently, keep distributing caresses and kisses over her belly, around the navel, never inside! On her hips, buttocks, inner thighs, exterior and interior lips, over her vagina. If you notice that she is sufficiently lubricated, you can begin to insert a finger very slightly. But only a little. Remember that the most sensitive part of the vagina is around the entrance. Then you can gently caress the clitoris. She will be showing you how much pressure to apply and the rhythm of the caresses. But keep in mind that this is not an orgasm. You are making love, and all these kisses and caresses are part of foreplay in lovemaking that will elicit the appropriate arousal.

ORAL SEX

I know that not everyone likes it, but if your aim is to get your partner to enjoy it, do not hesitate for a moment. Very gently at first run your tongue over her outer lips.

Open her vagina a little with your hand and gently suck the inner lips and muscles of the vagina. Gently press the tip of your tongue on her vagina. After that, you can move to the clitoris. The intensity of the pressure and the pace you follow should be set by her. I will tell you that when you give her oral sex, it is called cunnilingus, and when she does it to you, it is called fellatio.

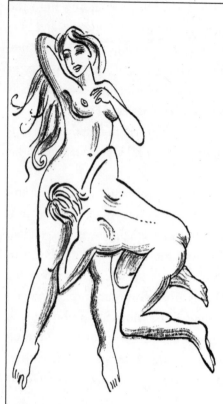

The position for oral sex can be quite varied. I will suggest two: her lying on her back with knees slightly bent, and you upside down with your head between her thighs; and you on your back and her "sitting" on your face, with her knees resting on the bed and her hands on the headboard. This second position facilitates movement for the woman, and she can guide your tongue toward the exact point where she wants to be stimulated.

I will tell you as a fact that oral sex is the surest way for a woman to reach an orgasm. In fact, some women do not get there with a partner, although they do through masturbation.

Penis-vulva caresses and penetration. The time has come for you to get in position to have intercourse. The penetration is close and the climactic moment too. First select the position in which you are going to start penetration. Or, rather, let her be the one who decides. At this point, agreeing is the easiest thing in the world. Once in place, and before entering her, stroke her genitals with the tip of your penis. If it was not erect enough, doing this will make you ready to explode. At this point, your partner's vulva is lubricated as an airplane engine, and just as ready for takeoff.

Penetrate her. The movements should be rhythmic, smooth, and steady. Occasionally stop for a moment, just to continue again. Try to gently caress her clitoris while moving. She will let you know if she likes it. Whisper in her ear what you feel. It will not be difficult; just let go. Forget that you are a tough, silent guy, and enjoy letting her know how you feel. What comes after this I cannot tell you, because not even the best poets have managed to express it. But if you have followed these steps thoroughly, I assure you, as the French say...*chapeau!*

SOME CONCRETE TECHNIQUES

If you read this chapter carefully, you do not need to know much more. But since I know you and I know that you like "details," I will provide some specific techniques that will take you and your partner to seventh heaven... Or beyond!

While you stimulate her clitoris with your tongue, insert two of your fingers—only halfway—in her vagina, with a smooth motion from the inside out.

Watch how she masturbates, and just before she reaches an orgasm, penetrate her gently. A simultaneous orgasm is guaranteed.

Use a feather to touch her genitals.

Place her clitoris between two of your fingers and stimulate her, without letting go, in a circular motion.

Place the palm of your hand on her mons pubis and, with a little pressure, move it up and down.

Insert two of your fingers in her vagina about an inch deep and press up a little. You will touch her G-spot. Move your fingers gently in a circular motion, and see what awaits you!

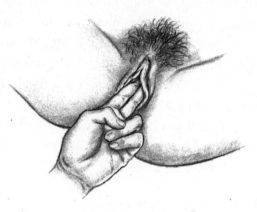

Secrete all the saliva you can. You can use a piece of gum if you want. With your wet tongue, lick around the entrance to the vagina.

Sex and fear

"I never had problems reaching an orgasm through masturbation, but the fear of getting pregnant inhibits me so much that I almost never get there when I make love with Ángel."

Julia, 22 years old

For centuries, sexuality and procreation have been inextricably linked. There were no really effective methods to prevent pregnancy, so every time a woman made love with a man, she ran the risk of getting pregnant. If you want to have a child, this chapter, for now, is not for you. But if this is not your case, and if, like me, you think that sex should not be for procreation only, you will agree that, in addition and above all, it is an almost inexhaustible source of play, pleasure, and communication. For this reason, the widest possible knowledge of the various contraceptive methods is essential to leading a sexual life free from fears and inhibitions. It is about enjoying your body and having wonderful orgasms. Remember that staying relaxed and stress-free is essential to having orgasms easily. So read, learn well, and select the method that best fits your situation.

THE IDEAL CONTRACEPTIVE METHOD

The truly ideal thing about contraceptive methods is the fact that they exist. Only since their emergence have women been able to enjoy sex freely. As to whether one is better than another, it is difficult to give a definitive answer, and, moreover, progress and new discoveries are made continually. The most appropriate method depends on each person and each situation. We will give an overview of the most common methods, and you can decide which one is ideal for you. Or the ideal ones—indeed, gynecologists recommend combining a few methods for total security.

Condom. Much has been said about the technological revolution and how it has changed society with computers, mobile phones, and everything else. But, for us, the most important revolution happened the day the condom was discovered. That wonderful little balloon that men put on before the sexual act—if it is well placed and you have checked the expiration date—is 100% secure because sperm does not reach the uterus. It is also unique when it comes to preventing sexually transmitted diseases. I have friends who complain that the condom feels unpleasant, or that it is a nuisance to stop to put it on just before starting. And I have known men who were reluctant to use it (of course, we never got to have sex). What matters is that it exists, and it is a great solution. It can even elicit a sexual game: try to put it on him, or choose condoms with different flavors—mmm, berry-flavored fellatio—or with those little ridges on the tip that caress particularly sensitive areas.

There are also female condoms. Many women consider them a good choice, especially if they do not have a steady partner.

Diaphragm. This is a kind of rubber cap that the woman inserts into her vagina to block access to the cervix. It should always be used together with a spermicidal. It is great for some, but it has a few drawbacks. If you intend on having a sexual relationship for the first time with someone you do not know well—that irresistible stranger who came on to you—it is not recommended. First, it is not effective in preventing STDs, and you have to wear it for 2 hours before having intercourse. Another drawback is that the first time you wear it, it should be put in place by a gynecologist; then you must ensure that you have it properly placed because misplacement can cancel its effect. However, it has the advantage that it does not cause hormonal changes in your body. Moreover, it "forces" you to have 2 hours—2 hours!—of foreplay prior to penetration. If your partner is willing to do the work, the result of those hours can bring you closer to paradise.

IUD. These small objects that a gynecologist introduces into your uterus are surprisingly effective, especially for women in stable, monogamous couples. They are placed inside you and can last for 5 to 10 years. Just like that! If you suffer frequent genital infections or have very heavy periods, this is not advisable. But this option offers many advantages: it does not have the side effects of hormonal methods, sex is not interrupted, it does not alter sensitivity, and it has been shown to protect against cervical and endometrial cancers. IUDs are very safe when it comes to preventing pregnancy, although they do not prevent STDs.

The pill. This pill, to be taken every day, at the same time, manages to block ovulation in your body, and therefore you cannot get pregnant. It is totally reliable. If you have painful periods, taking the pill for a time can be good for you. The new generation of pills has remarkably reduced some annoying side effects, such as weight gain or mood swings. But the biggest problem with this method is still the same: "forgetfulness." If you miss just one dose, its safety is not guaranteed. There are different types, so it is more appropriate for the gynecologist to point out the best option for you. None of them help prevent STDs.

Morning-after pill. For emergencies only! If you could not resist and you had intercourse without using any protection, it is possible to take this pill within 72 hours after intercourse. It contains a high dose of hormones that prevents the fertilized egg from getting implanted in the uterus. It can be provided to you as an outpatient. But be careful, because the amount of estrogen and progesterone in it is very large, so you should use it only when it is a real emergency.

Rhythm method. This is to have "full" intercourse—and who would want it incomplete?—only on those days in which the woman is not fertile, bearing in mind that the most fertile period is four days before and four days after the fourteenth day of the cycle. Another way to find out is by taking the vaginal temperature, but there are big differences from one woman to another, and taking the temperature of the vagina is rather cumbersome. No wonder they say the world is full of "children of the rhythm method..."

Hormonal injection. This consists of injecting into the body synthetic progesterone that prevents pregnancy. The advantage is that if you have problems remembering and forget to take the pill every day, with this method you only have to remember to get an injection every 2 months or so. The drawback is that it can have some side effects, like heavy periods and sometimes even weight gain.

Subcutaneous implants. A specialist places them under the skin of your arm, and these implants act by releasing progesterone. They last 5 years, and then they must be removed and replaced. Very few women have presented skin irritation or rejection of this method.

Contraceptive patches. They are small, squared, flesh-colored adhesive patches, which are placed in an area of the body that is not too visible (arms, shoulders, buttocks, or abdomen). They work like the pill, with the advantage that you only have to remember to wear them three times a month, because one is placed each week, and the fourth week you are off. If you are a smoker, are older than 32, are overweight, or have poor blood circulation, this method is not for you.

Vaginal ring. It consists of a transparent, flexible plastic ring that is placed as though it were a tampon. Its great advantage over the diaphragm is that you do not need to wear it in a precise way, because it releases hormones that pass directly into the bloodstream through the vaginal walls. It is a practical and effective method, and you must remember to put it in only once a month and take it off during the third week.

Tubal ligation. More than birth control, this is a life-long decision. If you have had the children you wanted, or if you have decided that motherhood is not for you, tubal ligation is a permanent solution to the issue of pregnancy. Neither the sperm nor eggs can go through, so it is impossible to get pregnant. The surgery is simple; the drawback is that, in most cases, there is no possibility of reversing it. If you are certain, it may be the perfect solution, but I would suggest that you think about it very carefully before doing this, because life takes many turns and you never know what may lie ahead.

Vasectomy. For us a vasectomy is perfect, because we have absolutely nothing to do. It is the man who has to undergo a minor operation to keep sperm from reaching the semen. The advantage over tubal ligation is that it is the man who has to undergo surgery, and especially if the circumstances change, in case you want to recover the ability to procreate, the chances of success are quite high. But if you have a steady partner and you are still hoping to have one or more children, you should not consider this method.

Coitus interruptus and other dangerous myths. This "method," other than being unique, consists of the man withdrawing his penis just at the "right time" and ejaculating outside the vagina. That is why it is also called "pulling out." Men tend to swear that they know how to do it, they have self-control, and you should not worry, but...watch out, friends! How can you be sure that your partner will be able to "pull out" precisely when he is enjoying himself the most? Moreover, prior to ejaculation, the penis secretes a fluid that may contain sperm. Do not even waste your time considering this very risky practice. It is also dangerous to have intercourse during menstruation, since sperm can survive up to 5 days, and if you ovulate right after you menstruate, pregnancy is possible.

A friend asked me, "What if I douche after intercourse, or I squat so that the semen does not reach the egg?"; another friend assured me that an infusion of blueberries with lemon zest applied as a plaster after intercourse was very effective. Douching, certain positions, all types of concoctions. Bullshit! None of it is true. Women tried for centuries and never got reliable results. If you do not want to get pregnant, you have only two options: abstinence—oh!—or using one of the methods that I have described to you.

SEXUALLY TRANSMITTED DISEASES (STDs)

In today's world, where sex is—fortunately—becoming freer and more frequent, and where changing partners is not strange, having some knowledge about STDs is absolutely essential. I do not intend to scare you. At this point in the book, you know me well enough to know that I am of the opinion that sex is a wonderful thing and we should try to get the most enjoyment out of it. However, some information about STDs will help you have safer, and therefore freer, and more enjoyable sexual relationships.

STDs are diseases that are transmitted from one person to another through sexual contact. However, for your peace of mind, I will say that all of them, including AIDS—although just partially—have a treatment and solution. Anyway, the best option for avoiding pregnancy as well as avoiding infection is prevention, and for this we just need to pay some attention and take necessary action. You must keep in mind that, with the exception of condoms, contraceptives do not work to prevent these diseases. Keep reading, and you will learn what are the most common STDs: their names, symptoms, treatment, and prevention.

Syphilis. Formerly known as the "French disease." Today it is on the decline, but for centuries it was a very serious disease, which can cause madness and, in many cases, death. Syphilis is caused by a virus called *Treoponema pallidum* that first inserts itself into the skin and then into the bloodstream. The first symptom is a kind of sore on the vagina, anus, or mouth. This "chancre," as it is called, appears approximately 1 month after having intercourse. As I said, today it has been virtually eradicated, and it is also easily treated.

Herpes. An infection that is also caused by a virus. The symptoms are a type of welts on the vulva or anus. They are very itchy and hurt when making love, so this condition is pretty easily identifiable. Also, it is usually accompanied by a slight fever. Specific treatment depends on the type of herpes, but it is always essential for the whole genital area to be very clean to keep the sores from becoming infected.

Gonorrhea. It is caused by bacteria, and its symptoms are very different in women than in men. Men who have gonorrhea experience pain when they urinate and expel a kind of pus from the penis. In women, the symptoms are much subtler: a little burning when urinating, flow a little thicker than usual and more yellowish in color, and a slight fever. As with syphilis, in our societies, where hygiene has become so widespread, this disease has almost completely disappeared. It is treated with antibiotics and does not leave any side effects.

Fungi. It is the most common and the least severe. You probably know someone who has had fungus somewhere in the body. Usually this occurs when the body's defenses are low for any reason, and the fungus causes some discomfort: itching in the vaginal area, flow that is somewhat thick and white and sometimes lumpy. It can be spread through sexual contact, but also by sharing underwear, towels, or clothes that come into contact with the genitals. Once detected, it can be treated easily and it disappears shortly thereafter. Both partners should be treated, because otherwise they immediately go back to being contagious.

AIDS. This is the most recent and also the most dangerous STD. It is spread through blood, semen, and vaginal fluid. It is brought on by a virus that attacks the sufferer's immune system. This means that the virus destroys the body's defenses. You have heard that some people are "carriers" but are not sick. What does it mean to be a "carrier"? It means that the AIDS virus is in the body but has not begun to act. This can last for years. Do you remember a basketball player named Magic Johnson? Years ago he declared he was a "carrier," and he is still out there doing talk shows. Once the virus starts to work, the body's defenses plummet, and the patient is more susceptible to all kinds of diseases. Until recently, AIDS was a fatal disease, but today there are very effective treatments. The treatment does not make it disappear entirely but keeps it under control, allowing the patient to live many years with it.

It must be very clear to you that AIDS only spreads in a very precise way (unprotected sex or sharing needles, usually). All that gossip that you can get it from pool water, saliva, or food are nothing but lies. Kissing poses no risk!

Although the picture looks a bit bleak, AIDS is actually very easily preventable. If your partner wears a condom, the risk disappears. It is as simple as that!

In general, the first essential preventive method, before other methods, is to have proper hygiene and regular doctor visits. The sexual organs are no different from other parts of the body. We must always keep them clean and in perfect condition. The opportunity may arise at any time! A daily shower and washing the genital area with soap and water before bed are more than enough under normal circumstances. Forget the special soaps and foreign substances. Simply use tap water and the same bath soap you use for the rest of the body.

It is essential that you visit the gynecologist every so often (twice a year at least) to check "the machine," perform the necessary exams and tests, and certify that it is fully prepared to "work."

In depth

"My relationship with Ernesto is superb. We make love frequently and I always have an orgasm, but sometimes I wonder: Is this it? Why not try something else?"

Miriam, 35 years old

By now, you know what to do to enjoy pleasurable orgasms. However, the world of sex is broad, rich, and varied, and its horizons are endless. In this chapter I suggest some more "exotic" techniques for exploring varieties of pleasure. As in sport, or art, sex can also go further, stronger, and higher.

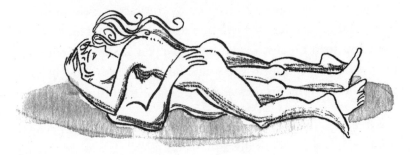

MULTIPLE ORGASMS

Any woman who has had an orgasm dreams of the possibility of having several of them consecutively. In fact, many women are not satisfied if they do not climax at least twice during sex. In laboratory experiments some women have demonstrated that it is possible to have 5, 10, and up to 25 orgasms separated by short intervals. Perhaps the latter is too much to ask...but why not try it? If after a single orgasm you do not feel satisfied, these pages will show you the way to have more.

First step. The key to experiencing multiple orgasms is to control the genital muscles. It has been shown that a woman's ability to contract and relax these muscles opens the door to reaching an orgasm more than once. Once, I attended an erotic show—yes, I am also curious about those shows—in which a woman smoked a cigarette with her vagina. Just as you hear it. Such was her control over her muscles that she inhaled and exhaled the smoke just as she would do with her own mouth, with the advantage that she never had a coughing fit!

Remember the "vaginal exercises" that were suggested in Chapter 1. And try to contract and relax the vaginal muscles until you get to feel them. You can help yourself by using the Ben Wa balls that we mentioned in the chapter on toys. Or, use a cucumber (peeled and carefully washed) that is not too large: insert it halfway into your vagina and hold it by contracting your muscles. With a bit of practice, you will be able to hold it in as long as you want and then expel it forcefully. Once you are able to contract the muscles for as long as you want and then let go, you will have taken the most important step toward having multiple orgasms.

Second step. If you have gained reasonable control of your genital muscles, it is time to put them to good use. When you are making love with your partner, use them to squeeze and release his penis while keeping pace with the rhythm of his movements. Do not panic if his moans make the windows rattle! Keep going until you feel close to having your first orgasm. When you are about to have an orgasm, relax your muscles and ask your partner to stop. Not to withdraw the penis from your vagina, but to stop moving until the sensation of an orgasm disappears. In that moment, ask him to start moving again, and do your contractions again until you feel the orgasm approaching. A moment before, stop again! I know it is not easy, but the rewards are really worth it. Begin again with the movements, and when you are about to climax, let go but contract your muscles with all your strength. The natural contractions of an orgasm will join this voluntary pressure, and you will have the longest and deepest orgasm of your life. With a little practice, it will extend until it lasts more than twice the duration of a normal orgasm.

If your partner has not yet finished, ask him to keep moving! Neither faster nor slower than before. At first you may not feel anything, but after 2 or 3 minutes, you will notice that orgasmic sensation reappear. Enjoy it! Contract the muscles as much as you can and enjoy. How long can you go on like this? Well, until you feel that you can do it no more. Or until your partner faints from pleasure from your muscle contractions.

SIMULTANEOUS ORGASMS

"I knew what it was to have an orgasm, and it gave me a feeling of fullness and intense pleasure. But when I had one at the same time as my partner, I felt as though the universe was giving me a hug."

Mónica, 27 years old

With a bit of technique you can have long, intense multiple orgasms, but wouldn't it be an even more beautiful experience to have them at the same time as your partner? This is probably the greatest pleasure we can experience in this world. If heaven exists, it should be something like this. Yes, sex is pleasure, fun, game. But it is also sharing and communicating with your partner, "getting lost" in him. I know nothing more sublime and deep than this feeling. Forgive me if I get poetic, but I am at a loss for words. If you have practiced the previous lessons, you probably already know that indescribable emotion. Now it is about your learning to do it whenever you want. Not all sexual relationships are the same, and you may not always feel like having an orgasm simultaneously. What is interesting is controlling the situation and getting there whenever you want. Do you always want it? Then pay attention.

First step. The secret to having a synchronized orgasm with your partner is knowing your own feelings. Therefore, the first thing to do is to learn them, step by step, on your own. You may think you know what happens in your body when you are about to climax. Do not be so sure. Sexual response is full of nuances and subtleties that make every relationship different. And that is why every one of them is so exciting!

The first step is to identify the stages your body goes through when you get excited, no matter the situation, place, or day of the week. Pay close attention to each of these stages, as if you were following a detailed city map to reach an exact location for an appointment. At what precise moment does your vagina lubricate? When does your breathing quicken? When does that intense tingling in your genitals begin? If you remember Chapter 1, your body goes through three distinct stages until you orgasm. Study these stages on your own, enjoying each one while you touch yourself. Now try to split them into shorter sequences to control them better. Although these sequences are different for each person, I suggest you identify these seven moments along the way:

1. You feel desire and begin to feel aroused.
2. Your vagina is already well lubricated.

3. You start to moan.
4. Tingling, loud moaning.
5. Pleasurable sensation in the genital area.
6. You are almost there.
7. Orgasm.

Each of these phases can be named so that you will remember them more easily. Familiarize yourself with them until you have perfectly identified them. I know it seems difficult, unnatural, and impossible to think of steps and sequences as your body quivers with pleasure. But take my advice. Try it; consider it a game. After a few sessions, reading the map of your feelings will be much easier than following the directions of a traffic cop. And the results will be very surprising.

Second step. Have you already established which stages your body goes through to reach an orgasm? Great! Now try to learn to control them, going from one to the next in order without skipping any. It is a simple exercise in concentration: focus your attention on each one, and try not to move to the next until you decide for yourself. At the third stage, are you no longer excited? Tap into your fantasies to get aroused again! Move faster! Breathe more heavily! Do you always skip the sixth stage? Think of something else! Relax your muscles more! You will see that it is fun and exciting. And it will help you know yourself and enjoy it more intensely. Soon you will completely control the phases of your arousal; you will know exactly where you are and when and how to move on to the next stage.

Third step. The moment of truth has arrived: the time to share your new knowledge with your partner. Tell him what you discovered, and encourage him to do the same. Since you already know what it is, at first you can guide him a little. Do you know how exciting it can be for the both of you to be able to control your arousal levels? With a bit of practice, you will find in this game an endless source of pleasure. It is important that the number of levels is the same for you both so that you will know at all times how things are going.

Once you are able to locate and control each step of the way, make love while keeping in mind what you know. It may not work the first time you try, or the second one, but who cares? It is not an exercise like lifting weights or doing crunches. The two of you will start to perfect the system, and you will continue to enjoy it in the meantime. What better way to learn something? At first, perhaps you might whisper, "I am at 4!" And he may giggle and go from 5 to 2. Help him return to 5 as soon as possible! You know what he likes, so do it! Over time you will learn to read each other's signs, and you will just have to press your head against the pillow for him to understand that 6 is about to arrive. Or you will understand that when he kisses you in that way, he is close to 7. It seems difficult, but you just need to trust each other and practice. And as the practice is so nice, it will not be difficult for you to repeat it over and over again, until you are both tired! When you both reach an orgasm at the same time, you will understand how much it was worth. And you will never forget how much fun it was to practice.

TANTRIC ORGASMS

"For me, sex has always been a very physical activity. Sure, I felt emotions and love, but that did not seem crucial, until I met Felipe, who had just arrived from India. He started talking to me about the spirit, and the truth is that I thought it was a bit boring. But when we made love, I loved it!"

Marisa, 34 years old

Everything that comes from the East has a special mystery: yoga, Kundalini energy, the Kama Sutra. In fact, there is a Latin saying,

Ex oriente, lux: "Wisdom comes from the East." How is this wisdom valuable once you are in bed? If you dare to experiment with tantric sex, you will find out for yourself. It is important to share these experiences with someone you trust completely, someone who wants to experience new things and venture into unknown territory.

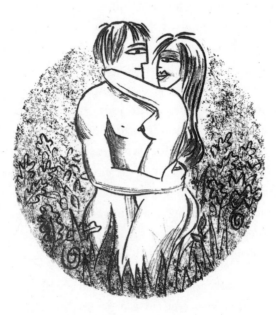

According to tantric tradition, sex has a strong spiritual component. And the aim of making love is to reach a cosmic orgasm and create a circle of energy that elevates the lovers over the material world, toward ecstasy and perfection. Sounds good, right? Try a tantric sex session with your partner one weekend.

Peace and harmony. You are going to need time and tranquility, so be very sure that no one will bother you. Unplug the phone and turn off the lights. A few candles—preferably red—will help create the right ambiance. You can also burn an incense stick if you like. After finishing the preparations, lay naked in bed without your bodies touching. Begin to gently caress each other, including the genitals, but without the intent of exciting one another mutually. This is most important! Do not start thinking that you would like to do this or that to your partner, or that you would rather have him kiss you passionately or caress your breasts. Try to keep your mind blank. After a while, the caresses will arouse you. Your sexual energies will start to run, starting from the genital area to a point located right at the center of the skull where the Kundalini, the most refined and pure energy, is concentrated. If you are already lubricated and your partner has an imposing erection, you are right on track. However, no outpourings! You still need to harmonize your breathing. Focus on your breathing and imagine that you inhale air from the vagina and breathe it out through your mouth, while your partner imagines that he draws air in through the mouth and exhales it through his penis. If the circle of sexual energy starts to overwhelm you, do not let it drag you. When your breathing is already harmonized, your vagina is lubricated, and his penis is erect, that will be the moment for penetration. In a comfortable position, let your partner insert his penis halfway into your vagina.

Stillness and ecstasy. At this point, you probably want to start moving like crazy. However, in tantric sex stillness is essential. Neither you nor your partner must move. Remain in the same position, with half of his penis in your vagina, and look into each other's eyes and continue with the visualization described above: take in air through your vagina and breathe it out through your mouth; your partner inhales through his mouth and exhales through his penis. Stay like this as long as you can. The only allowed movement is that which you are able to perform with your genital muscles but without using your hips at all. You are taking part in the cycle of sexual energy, the primal and creative energy. When you realize it, you will have one of the deepest orgasms of your life.

ANAL SEX

"I love to practice anal sex with my partner. It is a completely different feeling, and it makes me feel wild and capable of anything."

Patricia, 37 years old

Not all women like to practice anal sex. The connotations that this part of the body has for most of us are not exactly sexual. However, I know many women who practice anal sex and enjoy it. The muscles around the anus are highly sensitive, and stimulating them can create intense and unexpected pleasure.

If you have never practiced anal sex, you should go step by step. It is not advisable to indulge in a sudden fit of passion, because you can do real damage. It is best to start in a relaxed and comfortable position. Lie on your side on the bed and bend your waist slightly to give your buttocks to your partner—some proposition! Use an alcohol-free lubricant to prevent irritation. Your partner should start caressing your vulva and clitoris and then your buttocks until you are excited. Then, with a well-lubricated finger, he can caress you around the anal opening, lubricating the entire area well. Keep in mind that the anal muscles are much stronger than those of the vagina, and they are unaccustomed to opening easily. When it looks as though you are ready, tell him to proceed and insert his finger up to the second knuckle and gently begin to move. The next step is the insertion of a second finger. Gently, your partner can move both fingers inside and out for a while. The first time, you can leave it at that and switch to a bit of oral sex, for example, to reach stage 4 (remember?) and then enjoy a long simultaneous orgasm.

In later sessions you can go forward a little more. After caressing the area and inserting two fingers (never forget the lube!), your partner can bring his penis closer. At first, he must insert only the tip and stay still. The feeling will be new and strange and possibly a little scary. Wait until you feel comfortable. Only then tell him to continue. How far? As far as you say. I have friends who can stand a huge penis in their anus, while others are extremely sensitive and immediately feel pain. Only you can know how far your body allows being penetrated. At this point, your partner may begin to move smoothly. If he is well lubricated, you will feel a strong excitement and desire to caress your clitoris. He can do it for you, or you can do it yourself. With a little practice, you will get a different and intense orgasm.

Some common questions. Anal sex is a relatively uncommon practice, and it is therefore normal that doubts arise. There is certainly nothing off or wrong, and if you find it exciting and pleasurable, do not hesitate to practice it. Whenever you want. Many women I know have asked me questions about it, and these are some of the most common:

Why do most men like it? My dear, men like to put it anywhere, for the simple reason that it stimulates the most sensitive part of the penis, located at the bottom of the glans, and they get to have an orgasm easily.

My partner likes it when I insert a finger in his anus when he is going to have an orgasm; does that mean he is a homosexual? Not at all. Like I said, the muscles around the anus are highly sensitive, and many men and many women feel great excitement when penetrated there. In fact, sex shops sell "anal cones" that are purchased not only by homosexuals.

Does it hurt? If you follow the advice I gave you a moment ago, no. However, it is imperative that you practice it with a man whom you trust, especially in the beginning. Penetration that is too abrupt can be quite painful. It is essential to do it gently and that your partner follow your instructions to stop whenever you are in discomfort.

Isn't it a little "dirty"? As I have said several times throughout this book, the only limits on your sexuality are those that you impose on yourself. Dirty? And who does not like to feel a little dirty, wild, or animal-like occasionally?

What is a black kiss? Well, this question is not as common, but since you have asked me, I will tell you that a black kiss is oral sex... on the anus.

VARIATIONS AND VARIANTS

"I love making love, and Daniel is great in bed... But what really drives me wild is doing it on the beach, behind a dune, and knowing that there are people nearby who could surprise us."

Laura, 35 years old

I will repeat it once again: limits? Only those your own imagination can impose. Sexuality is virtually unlimited. Do you want to find new ways to enjoy sex? Do you want to "deepen" your sexual relationship with your partner? We have reviewed a number of alternatives to the typical 10-minute "marital" sex, but, of course, the catalog is far from over. Explore things outside of the routine. For example, if you always shower before making love, go to bed after sunbathing for hours, when your sweat runs down your crotch and your breasts appear to be bathed in olive oil. If you like slow and restful sex, practice it when you have 10 minutes before you are late for work. If you always do it in your room, why not try it in the kitchen or bathroom? A friend used to tell me that her husband was not very fiery and seemed bored with sex. They used to make love only before bedtime or before getting up on weekends. One night, she woke him up by stroking his penis at 4:00 in the morning. Since then, every time we talk about our respective sex lives, my friend sighs and looks out into space.

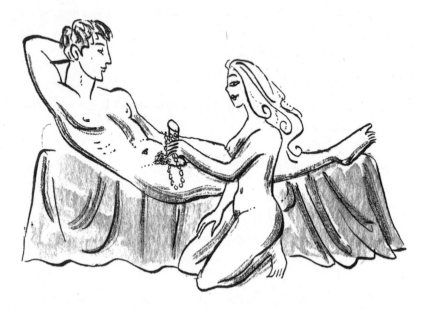

A little curiosity, an open mind, and great confidence in your partner are enough to deepen your sexual relations. Try some of these ideas when you feel like innovating your sexual encounters:

Rent a pornographic movie and learn the script. They are usually very simple, and it will not take a lot of work. When your partner comes home, play the video and try to re-create the dialogue.

Explore the tantric orgasm: try seven brief halfway penetrations. Then a long and deep one.

Wait for him naked to get home from work. It is a provocative and exciting way to get his sexual attention.

Ask him to pour a glass of champagne on your clitoris. You can imagine what follows.

Play with an ice cube as it begins to melt. You can rub yourselves with it, and then run your tongue wherever you want.

On your genitals, apply vanilla ice cream and try to do a "sixty-nine."

Play "everything is allowed minus penetration" until you both have an orgasm.

Doubts, questions, and testimonials

Does your mind wander while making love? Does your partner have an orgasm so quickly that it barely gives him time to have intercourse? Did you like it when he tied your hands to the bed, but you are afraid it might be a perversion? Are you unsure how AIDS is spread exactly? If you still have doubts and questions, or you just do not feel satisfied with your relationships, this is your chapter.

DOUBTS AND QUESTIONS

Premature ejaculation. *"My partner has an orgasm almost immediately. I barely touch his genitals and he gets so excited that he ejaculates even before penetration; what can I do?"*

Your case is much more common than you think. Men have sex on their minds almost all the time, and sometimes it just takes a suggestive look for them to shudder with pleasure. That makes them suffer. And we end up suffering. Fortunately, there is a solution. If he manages to enter you before ejaculating, you can use the "pause" technique to stop any movement seconds before climax, without removing his penis from your vagina. After a while, you can start gently moving again. If his case is so severe that he ejaculates before penetration, you must use the "gripping" technique: when he is about to ejaculate, hold his glans and press it firmly at the bottom to stop the flow of semen. He may lose his erection, but he will recover quickly. With a little practice, he will get better control over his ejaculations. And you both will be happier and satisfied.

SUBMISSION

"When Felipe suggested tying my hands to make love, I did not think it was a great idea. I agreed because he promised to behave delicately... And I must say it was a delight to be immobilized while being touched. On another occasion I was the one who tied him... It was a super exciting experience to have my guy fully available to my wishes. I also blindfolded him...and I still quiver when I remember his moans of pleasure."

As I have said several times, any manifestation of sex is as good and natural as the others. It is not recommended that you let just anyone handcuff you. But if you trust your partner and you are sure that he will not go too far without asking prior permission, go ahead and practice as much as your body desires!

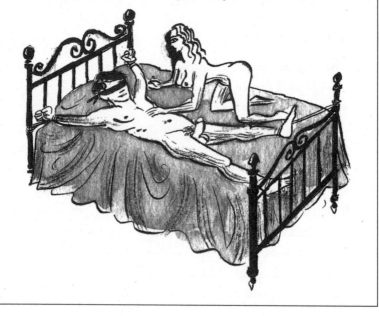

Does he enjoy it with me? *"My partner always reaches an orgasm when we make love, but sometimes I'm not sure if he enjoys it. Asking him seems a little rude."*

I advise you to reverse the question: do you enjoy it with him? Women often give too much—or all—importance to whether the man enjoys it. Don't you think that if he makes love to you whenever possible, he has to like it? Despite their boasting, men are quite shy when it comes to talking about sex with women. And they tend to keep quiet during and after lovemaking. Some would even feel humiliated if they were to admit to having enjoyed themselves as never before. In this case, I recommend that you be indirect yet straightforward: the next time you make love, tell him how wonderful it was and what a great lover he is. Give details; tell him how good you felt when he caressed your breasts. Hopefully, he will also be able to express himself more freely.

Vibrator. *"Several friends have told me how exciting it is to use a vibrator, but it still embarrasses me."*

And why are you ashamed? The vibrator is an absolutely harmless gizmo used to spend delightful moments. I know many women who use it and masturbate to full satisfaction. It hardly makes any noise, it does not stain, it does not get tired at the ideal time…it is a dream! I only recommend that you not use it for penetration. It is more pleasant for stimulating your clitoris and other parts of the body. Find a rather small one to carry in your bag without problems. If you trust your partner, suggest that you use it during lovemaking. When the time comes for penetration, get on top of him, and as you move with his penis in your vagina, tell him to caress your clitoris with the vibrator. Then you will not want to do anything else!

Premenstrual syndrome. *"In the days before menstruation I do not want to make love. Am I sick?"*

Many women feel a little weird in the days before menstruating. Some feel that their breasts are swollen and they seem more irritable than usual. If you do not want to make love during those days, try to have sexual relations that do not include penetration. Oral sex or masturbation can provide you with more pleasurable orgasms. And I assure you that your sex life will be more enriched. Talk to your partner about this. Caress him and guide his hand to where you most like.

AIDS. *"I thought it was impossible to contract AIDS through oral sex; am I wrong?"*

Yes, you are wrong. AIDS can be transmitted through blood, semen, and vaginal fluid. So, if you practice fellatio on your partner and his semen gets in your mouth, there is a risk of contagion. The same applies if he gives you cunnilingus: your vaginal fluid will reach his throat. With regard to AIDS, it is recommended that you and your partner get tested. It is a simple blood test, and any hospital will do it for free. In these times, you need to be sure. And, therefore, always use a condom if you make love to strangers. Sex is to be enjoyed, and no shadow of suspicion should darken the horizon.

Changing positions. *"My partner asks me to change positions many times while making love. And I almost always lose my arousal with so many changes. What do I do?"*

You are not the only one! Men think they impress us by changing positions and choreography. And they are convinced that in doing so, we consider them more desirable.

There is nothing special in getting distracted before such skill deployments. Help your partner relax and forget his alleged feats, for instance, by touching each other. The important thing is to make him "see" what you enjoy, literally: show him with your body and with your gestures how you have an orgasm. When he contemplates you in that wonderful state, he will forget his athletic "prowess" and try to do what it really takes for you to experience that again.

Ménage à trois. *"My boyfriend has asked me to bring a friend to make love with us. I do not dislike the idea, but I have my doubts. What do you recommend?"*

In erotic films, it is very common to see several actors making love together. Of course, real life is not a movie, but why not try it sometime? It is essential that you do it only if you are sure of it. If you do it to please him, but you do not find it appealing, it is likely that the experience will be a complete failure. Now, if, as you say, you do not dislike the idea, forget your doubts! Playing with two bodies at once, instead of the same old thing, may be very exciting.

Ridiculous. *"I cannot help it. When I have my partner's head between my legs, I feel so ridiculous that I start to laugh and I cannot feel anything."*

Laughter is good therapy for almost anything, but in this situation? This position is really a bit strange, especially if he is going bald. But the solution is not difficult to find. Focus on your feelings. Hold his head in your hands and set the pace of his movements. After a few seconds, you will be so comfortable that your fear of ridicule will have disappeared. And if you laugh, there will be other reasons for it: some orgasms are so pleasurable that it is impossible not to laugh.

HE WILL NOT LIKE ME

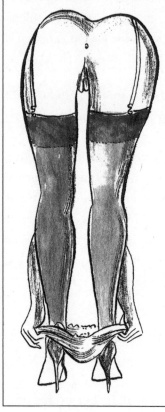

"I don't like making love with the light on because I'm sure that if he sees me naked, he will not like me."

As I said in Chapter 2, a woman is rarely ugly for a man if she is naked and wants sex. They are so absorbed in what awaits them that they do not usually notice the details. While you convince yourself, light colorful candles and put on some sexy clothes. How about taking off all your clothes but leaving your stockings, suspender belts, and heels? The image of your panties sliding down your legs, while leaving your private parts exposed, will drive him crazy with excitement... And why not? Wear that sexy outfit while you make love. This scene will become material for his erotic fantasies and memories.

Masturbation. *"I've masturbated since a young age and I've always felt good, but I get the feeling that my current partner is not amused by the idea. What do I do? Should I give up?"*

I hope you are referring to giving up on your partner. Masturbation is perfectly natural, pleasant, convenient, and even healthful. And nobody has the right to interfere in such personal matters. Ideally you should try to show him how nice it is to masturbate. You can try touching him, and teaching him to do the same for you. When you see pleasure on his face, his scruples will disappear.

Gynecologist. *"It seems a bit stupid, but I'm embarrassed to go to the gynecologist because I think he will notice that I masturbate."*

Have you ever thought that gynecologists do not give a damn whether you masturbate or not? When you go to the doctor for a checkup or because you do not feel well, you expect a treatment or a remedy for your situation—not for him to investigate exactly how you touch your clitoris. But just so you will remain calm: there is no way a gynecologist would know whether you masturbate or not—unless you tell him.

SOME COMPLAINTS

"Why is there so much to know and so much effort in order to enjoy sex? Isn't it something natural?"

Nothing prevents you from having sex without knowing absolutely anything about your genitals, or the importance of masturbation, or the role of fantasy... But then do not complain if you do not have an orgasm! A friend of mine always says that making love without an orgasm hurts. Perhaps she exaggerates a bit, but if you do not know where the clitoris is, and do not know the risks of AIDS transmission, or you are not interested in feeling attractive and desirable to your partner, your sexual relations will soon fall into the routine, and your orgasms will hardly come with the speed and intensity you want. Do not be lazy! Read at least one book about sex every year, mind your appearance, and explore the feelings that give you pleasure. It is never too late to start. Your sexuality will be enriched, you will enjoy life more, and the world will seem a much more beautiful place. You will be much happier.

"I never have fantasies while making love with Carlos. It would seem to me as a kind of infidelity."

Have you ever wondered if your partner fantasizes about other women? Have you seen his expression when he sees Sharon Stone taking off her clothes in a movie? Do you think that he is then thinking about the bank account? Is he cheating for that? Make no mistake! Fidelity is a very serious issue that every couple should determine in their own way, but, of course, it has nothing to do with fantasizing! As Chapter 5 says, having certain fantasies does not mean we want them to be fulfilled. My friend Amelia, who just turned 40, told me, "When I finally realized the importance that fantasies lend to reaching an orgasm, I began to imagine many times that I practiced anal sex, and that excited me much. One night, Jesús and I tried it. And it was a disaster! I did not like it; it was anything but sexy. However, when we make love, I keep imagining scenes of anal sex, and I find them very exciting."

"I never have an orgasm with a man. I enjoy kissing and fondling, but only climax by masturbating."

Now that you have read this book, be prepared to get there! An orgasmic woman, and you are one, is "always" orgasmic. Do men move too fast? Do they finish before you have a chance to get aroused? Do they not touch you in the right places? Teach them! When you are with a man, show him the way, tell him what you like, get in the proper position so that his movements stimulate you where you find it most enjoyable, and masturbate while he moves inside you. Listen to what Alejandro told me: "When Martha and I make love and she is on top of me, my eyes enjoy her entire body. I can see how my penis enters her vagina. I love watching her breasts swaying, and I run over her body with my hands. I squeeze her buttocks, or I rub her belly, or explore her clitoris, and with my fingers, I feel my penis rubbing her vagina. But what really drives me wild is her facial expression as she touches herself and starts to have an orgasm."

"I had an orgasm the first time I made love, but since then I only have them occasionally."

Orgasms are part of our nature. Sex attracts us in such an intense way because we expect reaching that climax of pleasure. You yourself know what it is, because you have felt it. What happens then? Why does it happen sometimes and not others? As always, the key is information. If you know exactly what happens to your body when you climax, if you know your sexual organs and their most sensitive spots and you feel ready and confident, orgasms will become commonplace. Natalia, 25, summed it up for me with these words: "I had an orgasm the first time I made love with my boyfriend. It is not strange because we were working up to it for 5 months before having full sexual intercourse. I was so excited that it did not take me long to climax. However, the following times it was not as easy. Sometimes I would and sometimes not. We both thought about it and started asking friends and reading books about sex. We learned a lot of things that we had no idea about. Now we try to make love whenever we can, because orgasms are sure to happen!"

"Making love for me is not very fun; I prefer to masturbate. When I'm with my partner, I dare not take the initiative because I think he likes it better that way."

Are you aware of what you are missing? We often have this idea that men like demure and passive women. We think that with a woman like that they feel more masculine and enjoy sex more. Nothing is further from the truth! In today's world, men are attracted to women who are active, who work, who take action, who know what they want. Listen to what Ricardo, a 35-year-old friend, said to me: "Like most men, I fantasize about women who are a little sexually aggressive, but most women I know are very shy about sex, do not like to talk about the subject, and when it comes to having intercourse, they are content with simply lying in bed. At one point, I even thought that women do not really like sex and only did it to please men. Then I met Fina, who loves sex. And not just because she cares about me, but because she enjoys it as much as I do. It's the best thing that could've happened to me."

TESTIMONIALS

One of the issues of most concern to women in long-term relationships is keeping sexual attraction alive. Since experience is always the best teacher, I asked all the happy couples I know what the trick is. Here are some of their responses:

"I think Armando continues to like me because I've never asked him if he likes me. I feel attractive, even if he does not tell me so. And that also gives me self-assurance. I try to take care of myself and stay fit: I exercise, follow a diet, dress up to go out. I never ask him if he wants to make love because if he likes me and I feel like it, why would he not want to? It seems obvious to me."

Arantxa, 29 years old

"My husband and I love surprises. When he least expects it, he gets home from work and finds me naked on the living room couch. 'Where are the children?' he asks alarmed. I've sent them to my sister's house. He approaches me, and I can tell by his expression that he has realized that the perfume I'm wearing is not the usual. He still hasn't been able to speak and is beginning to show signs of excitement. Then I start to undress him slowly, starting with his pants. Before touching his penis, I unbutton his shirt. What happens next depends on the moment, and the best part is that we never know who will surprise whom. Sometimes the

surprise takes weeks to arrive, and other times several days in a row. We both stay alert, knowing that, at any time, we could end up fucking like crazy."

Consuelo, 43 years old

"Javier and I had been living together for more than 10 years. At first everything was wonderful, but over time our sex life started getting cold. Not that I did not have orgasms, but the two of us started to show less interest. I got worried because I was afraid that making love was starting to become something of a formality. Then a friend lent me a book on tantric sex. What a discovery! I spoke with Javier, and at first he was a bit skeptical. But one day I convinced him, and we gave it a try. Wow! The both of us there, facing each other, naked, trying not to think about sex and caressing each other by candlelight... It was fascinating! Since then, when I think of formalities, I just remember those at the bank. Sex now fills our lives even more than when we met."

Irene, 38 years old

"We use the technique of the 'ideal night.' We have normal intercourse whenever we want, but each week one of us, taking strict turns, proposes an ideal night. It does not need to be a fixed day. Rather, it depends on our inspiration. What does it consist of? Well, there's the catch. The one in charge that week proposes anything that comes to mind, and the other has to agree to it. The only condition is for no one to get hurt. I'm a little embarrassed to confess this, but I've discovered some things that if someone were to tell me about them, I wouldn't believe them. I would've never figured out that anal sex was so exciting! Or that José Luis enjoys it when his hands are tied behind his back. One day he showed up with a vibrator, and since then it has become a regular part of our games. It's priceless!"

Nazareth, 31 years old

Now what?

If you have read the book carefully and you have followed my advice, I am sure you have been able to have easier, longer, and more intense orgasms than before. However, whether you have a steady partner or you have casual sex, life never fails to offer new incentives to fully enjoy your sexuality, as well as new difficulties.

Banish the routine. I know you come home tired from work, and you have to clean around the house and maybe take care of the children. But if you allow the routine to overpower you, and the only thing you do is watch TV and go to sleep right after, life will end up looking monotonous.

Why should it be any different with sex? If you always do it in the same position, at the same time, and in the same place, even if everything works well, more or less, sooner or later you will get bored. Do you not make small changes in your work to make it more bearable? Do you not change the furniture occasionally to give your home a different ambiance? Why then do you not do that with sex? In the end, this is the most pleasant road to happiness. Review the suggestions in Chapter 8. Here are a few more:

Sit naked with your partner on the living room carpet in front of a bowl of peeled shrimp or clams and feed each other.

Buy yourself a vibrator and use it with your partner next Monday. Yes, only if it is Monday!

Suggest that you go for a walk out in the countryside. That day put on a long skirt and no underwear. Once you are in a secluded spot, ask him to lie down on the grass, open his fly, and, without removing your clothes, sit on his penis and gently put him inside you. It will be very exciting to make love surrounded by nature... Also, if someone should walk by, you can pretend that you are just listening to the sound of birds.

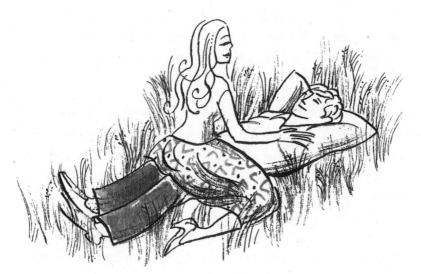

The next time you go on vacation, give yourselves a bath at sunset. Start stroking him underwater. Be sure that it is in a place where you have some stability!

Make an effort. Enjoying sex requires time and attention. Besides the fact that we are not born knowing, you can always learn more. Read books with your partner about sex. Or read them yourself and share your discoveries with him. Leaf through magazines; watch movies. It is not about your doing this every day. Who has time for that? But, occasionally, treat yourself and look for that article you were told about or rent that movie in the video store. Your effort will not be in vain.

Feel pretty! Remember that you are attractive. And do not wait for your partner to tell you so. Exercise, be mindful of the calories, make sure your skirt fits snugly around the hips, and go get a haircut... Feel pretty! You are an orgasmic being, and you will continue to be so for as long as you want. One of my nephews told me that he once caught his grandmother masturbating and froze. But why not? Sexuality has no age, nor does beauty. It is not a matter of opinion, but of attitude. If you like yourself, others will like you!

Precious time. Today we live in a world of haste and stress in which it seems that there is never time for anything. However, if you stop for a moment, you will realize that you actually waste time on activities that do not interest nor satisfy you. Your sexual relationships require that you dedicate to them a portion of that precious time. And you do not need to go very far to find the motivation. Is there anything that makes you feel healthier than an orgasm? On the bus, at work, at home alone, in those brief moments of leisure that are often wasted, think about sex. Imagine, fantasize, and exercise your vaginal muscles.... You may not have to wait until you go to bed to enjoy once more.

Glossary

AIDS. Acquired immunodeficiency syndrome, an STD that causes progressive weakening of the body's defense system. The acronym AIDS is how it is known in many places, especially on the Internet.

Amenorrhea. Lack of menstruation.

Anovulatory. Substance that impedes ovulation and, therefore, pregnancy.

Ben Wa balls. Metal or latex balls that are inserted into the vagina to tone muscles and produce excitement.

Bisexual. A person who has sex with people of both genders.

Cervix. Part of the uterus that connects it to the vagina.

Chancre. Type of hard, painless sore caused by syphilis; appears in the vagina, anus, or mouth.

Clitoris. Essential genital organ in female sexuality. It is located above the urethra, or opening where urine is expelled, and it is covered by something like a hood. It is erectile like a man's penis.

Coitus interruptus. Latin term used to describe an ineffective birth control method that involves removing the penis from the vagina before the ejaculation occurs.

Condom. Balloon-shaped contraceptive. Generally made out of latex and molds to the shape of the penis. It prevents sperm from reaching the cervix. There are also female condoms, although that is a more recent and less widespread method.

Contraception. All methods used to prevent pregnancy.

Contraceptive injection. (See anovulatory) Anovulatory contraceptive that consists of supplying a large amount of hormones. It is applied approximately every 2 months. It may have side effects.

Contraceptive pill. Hormonal contraception that is very reliable but requires constancy and memory, as it must be taken each day for a period of 21 days.

Cunnilingus. Latin expression used to refer to the stimulation of the female genitals with the mouth.

Cystitis. Bladder infection that causes irritation and painful urination.

Diaphragm. Contraceptive "barrier" that prevents sperm from reaching the uterus. The first time, it must be placed inside the vagina by a gynecologist. It must be precisely placed 2 hours before sex, and then removed.

Ejaculation. Expulsion of seminal fluid or semen through the penis.

Embryo. Name given to the fertilized egg during the first 3 months of pregnancy.

Endometrium. Wall membrane of the uterus where the fertilized egg is implanted. Each month, if there is no pregnancy, it detaches along with other substances and it is expelled through the vagina. This expulsion is usually called "menstruation" or "a period."

Erection. Hardening and enlargement of the penis or clitoris. It is caused by increased blood flow to these areas during sexual arousal.

Fallopian tubes. Ducts that connect the ovaries to the uterus or womb. Through them the egg travels, and fertilization occurs in them.

Fellatio. Stimulation of the penis with the mouth.

Fertile days. Time when women's ovulation occurs and pregnancy is therefore likely. Includes days 10 through 18 of the cycle.

Fertilization. Union of a sperm and an egg.

Fetus. Name given to the embryo after the third month of pregnancy.

Genital herpes. STD that causes inflammation of the genital organs and pain during intercourse.

Genitals. Group of organs that are involved in sex and reproduction.

Glans penis. Tip of the penis.

G-spot. Sort of large mole or protrusion located on the anterior wall of the vagina, about two or three centimeters from the entrance. It is extremely sensitive, and its stimulation is accompanied by great sexual excitement.

Hormonal implants. Subcutaneous implants that release hormones that inhibit pregnancy. They are placed for 5 years.

Hormone. Chemical substance that regulates the functioning of organs and the body in general.

Hymen. Membrane that partially protects the entrance to the vagina. Commonly called "virgo."

Intercourse. Sexual encounter that includes penetration.

IUD (intrauterine device). Contraceptive consisting of a small piece of plastic that the gynecologist places inside the uterus for a period of 5 to 10 years.

Labia majora. Also called "external labia." Folds of skin surrounding the vulva to protect it.

Labia minora. Folds of skin that protect the vagina, urethra, and clitoris. Located below the labia majora, they are also called "inner labia."

Latex. Material increasingly used to manufacture many items related to sex: condoms, Ben Wa balls, anal cones, and others.

Libido. (See *sexual desire*)

Masturbation. Self-stimulation of the sex organs to have an orgasm. Often done with the hands, but different objects may be used.

Menstrual cycle. Interval of time from the first day of your period until the first day of the next period. Its duration varies from woman to woman, but it is always around 28 days.

Menstruation. Blood flow that is expelled through the vagina. Occurs once a month due to shedding of the endometrium and other substances from the uterine lining if pregnancy has not occurred.

Mons pubis. Female genital area covered with hair.

Morning-after pill. A hormonal compound administered after risky sex. It must be taken within 72 hours after intercourse and used only in case of an emergency.

Ovaries. Female sex glands that produce the eggs. Located on the sides of the uterus, to which they are linked through the fallopian tubes.

Ovulation. Process of formation and release of the egg from the ovary toward the uterus through the fallopian tubes. Coincides with the days of maximum fertility for the woman.

Ovum. Female sex cell.

Patch. Small adhesive square that sticks to the skin and acts as a contraceptive, releasing hormones that are absorbed through the skin and enter the bloodstream.

Pelvis. Area of the body located on the lower abdomen.

Penis. Male genitalia. It consists of body and glands. In idle status it is limp and flexible. When it is erect due to sexual arousal, it enlarges and stiffens.

Period. (See *menstruation*)

Plateau. One of the phases of an orgasm.

Pregnancy. Implantation of an ovum fertilized by a sperm in the endometrium, located in the walls of the uterus.

Premature ejaculation. Ejaculation that occurs before it is desired.

Premenstrual syndrome. Light mental and physical changes that occur in some women in the days before menstruation.

Pulling out. (See *coitus interruptus*)

Rhythm method. Contraceptive method named after its discoverer. It is related to the temperature of the vagina, and it is scarcely reliable.

Scrotum. A type of skin pouch that holds the testicles.

Semen. Milky-white liquid that carries sperm. Secreted by the testes.

Sexual desire. Also called "libido." Impulse that leads us to want to have sex with another person.

Sexually transmitted disease (STD). Disease that is transmitted through sexual contact. Penetration is not necessary to occur, since it can also be transmitted through oral sex.

Sperm. (See *semen*)

Spermatozoid. Male sex cell. The testes produce it. Travels in the semen through the vagina and cervix to fertilize the egg.

Spermicides. Substances that kill sperm. Often used in the form of gel or jelly to complement other contraceptives.

STD. (See *sexually transmitted disease*)

Syphilis. STD that is virtually eradicated today, although very serious and widespread in the past. Today it is easily cured with penicillin. The first symptom is a sore (see *chancre*) in the vagina, anus, or mouth.

Testicles. Male glands that produce sperm.

Transsexual. Person who feels as though he or she belongs to the opposite gender.

Transvestite. Person who wears clothes of the opposite gender.

Tubal ligation. Radical and definitive method of contraception. Consists of cutting the tubes to prevent the egg from meeting with sperm, thus preventing fertilization and pregnancy.

Urethra. Tube that connects the bladder to the outside of the body. It is used to expel urine and, in the case of men, also to expel semen.

Uterus. Female genital organ where the pregnancy develops. In its walls is the endometrium, which is where the egg will remain once fertilized.

Vagina. Tube that connects the vulva to the uterus. The penis enters it during intercourse.

Vaginal discharge. Lubricating and protective substance secreted in the vagina.

Vaginal ring. Clear plastic ring that is placed in the vagina and serves as a hormonal contraceptive.

Vasectomy. Radical contraceptive method that consists of surgical intervention to prevent semen from containing sperm.

Vulva. Female sexual organ including the mons pubis, the labia, the clitoris, and the tip of the woman's urethra.